BLUEPRINT

BUILD A BULLETPROOF
BODY FOR EXTREME
ADVENTURE IN 365 DAYS

ROSS EDGLEY

BLUEPRINT

HarperCollins*Publishers*

HarperCollins*Publishers*
1 London Bridge Street
London SE1 9GF

www.harpercollins.co.uk

HarperCollins*Publishers*
1st Floor, Watermarque Building, Ringsend Road
Dublin 4, Ireland

First published by HarperCollins*Publishers* 2021

10 9 8 7 6 5 4 3 2 1

Text © Ross Edgley 2021
Diagram illustrations by Liane Payne © HarperCollins*Publishers* 2021
Exercise illustrations by Ben Hasler/NB Illustration

Ross Edgley asserts the moral right to be identified as the author of this work

A catalogue record of this book is available from the British Library

HB ISBN 978-0-00-848703-4
TPB ISBN 978-0-00-848704-1

Printed and bound in the UK using 100% renewable electricity at CPI Group
(UK) Ltd

MIX
Paper from
responsible sources
FSC
www.fsc.org **FSC™ C007454**

This book is produced from independently certified FSC™ paper to ensure
responsible forest management.

For more information visit: www.harpercollins.co.uk/green

CONTENTS

I feel so lucky to have had an incredible career as an athlete, adventurer and author, and I feel privileged to be coached and mentored by some of the greatest minds in sports science. But I want to specifically dedicate this book to two of my greatest teachers, Richard and Jacqueline Edgley (also known as Mum and Dad). You've been there for every mountain climbed, ocean swum and degree studied, and without you this book simply wouldn't exist.

FOREWORD

By Eddie 'The Beast' Hall, World's Strongest Man in 2017

Without a shadow of a doubt Ross Edgley is the craziest bastard – sorry, athlete – I know. Coming from me, that's saying something.

Although the world knows him for swimming 1,780 miles around Great Britain, climbing a rope the height of Everest (8,848 m) or doing a triathlon while carrying a 100 lb tree for charity, very few people understand the sheer number of hours he dedicates to research and training to make it all possible. As a friend and training partner I do, and have even witnessed (and endured) his brutal training sessions first-hand. Whether it be swimming ice miles across a frozen lake, running 10 km barefoot across snow and ice or pushing a one tonne tractor across a field for 10 hours in the middle of winter wearing nothing but a skimpy pair of swimming trunks, believe you me, Ross is not scared of a challenge.

In the pursuit of excellence, it's often said there's a fine line between genius and insanity. As the World's Strongest Man in 2017 and the first person to deadlift 500 kg, I understand what it takes to push your body beyond what people think is possible. But while I've done this within the realms of extreme strength, Ross has done it within the world of extreme endurance, and I recognise it requires a very specific and unique mindset. This is a mindset that Ross brilliantly describes with 100 per cent honesty and transparency in this book, blending elite sports science with theory, philosophy and some genuine originality.

For me, that's why this book is so pioneering. It's the first of its kind to show the inner workings of a sports science genius. Once you begin to understand the theory and psychology behind it, you begin to understand Ross. You start to realise there is method to the madness and, above all else, you understand how he built a level of endurance that verges on superhuman.

Essentially, this book is for anyone wanting to push themselves out of their comfort zone, achieve a goal and upgrade their training to another level – often getting very cold, very tired and very hungry in the process.

PART 1 |
WHY WE
ADVENTURE

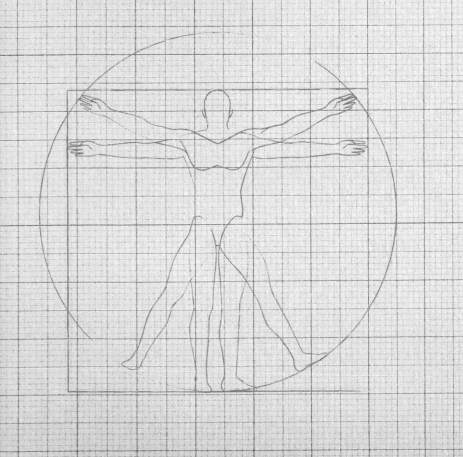

Every human should learn *Why We Adventure*.

For some, this comes naturally as the desire is innate and wired into our DNA. Research shows a proportion of the population are born with a variant of the DRD4 gene (known as DRD4-7R) that makes us genetically predisposed to take risks and travel with a restless curiosity.[1] More commonly referred to as the 'wanderlust gene', it's believed people who possess this genetic code have lower sensitivity to dopamine (our feelgood hormone) and therefore require a bolder and braver lifestyle to satisfy their biological make-up.

This partly explains why we Homo sapiens migrated from Africa over 50,000 years ago and then continued to colonise the entire world some 20,000 years ago. Scientists believe our wanderlust gene-carrying ancestors were the ones who pioneered this exploration of our planet as they climbed mountains, crossed oceans and had dreams of exploring beyond the horizon.

But what about those without the wanderlust gene?

Well, I would argue they also need adventure (perhaps more so). Yes, granted they're not inherently programmed with a desire to feel the sand beneath their toes in the Sahara Desert or go streaking in the snow across the Arctic Circle, but they require adventure to escape the shackles of the 'comfort zone'. Defined as, 'Behavioural space where your activities and behaviours fit a routine and pattern that minimises stress and risk' the comfort zone is also a place where ambition and creativity come to die.

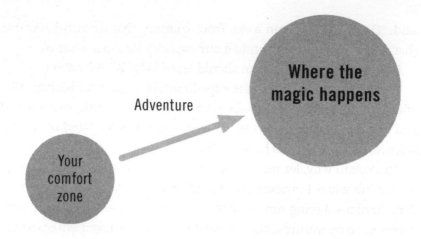

Although stress often comes with negative connotations, science shows a small dosage in our lives can often be a good thing as a catalyst for growth and provides a powerful motivation to act. This is based on the work of Hungarian physician Hans Selye (1950) who stated certain stress, which he called eustress (from the Greek prefix *eu-* meaning 'good'), can be a motivating force to move faster, further and into uncharted territory where lives are enriched by new experiences. In fact, this type of stress empowers you to grow in three areas:

1. **Emotionally.** Eustress can result in positive feelings of contentment, inspiration and motivation.
2. **Psychologically.** Eustress helps us build our self-efficacy, autonomy and resilience.
3. **Physically.** Eustress helps us build our body (e.g. through completing a challenging workout).

But without eustress, we fail to leave our comfort zone. As a result, we atrophy valuable attributes of creativity, courage and valour. This is why the famous Swiss author and adventurer Ella Maillart said, 'One travels to run away from routine, that dreadful routine that kills all imagination and all our capacity for enthusiasm.'

In summary, every human should learn Why *We Adventure*.

Yes, maybe not a large-scale expedition, but (whether biologically wired or not) everyone needs a small serving of risk, excitement and eustress within the great outdoors for reasons related to sports science, psychology and philosophy.

To explain why, let me share a story that had a profound impact on my life when I crossed the Arctic Circle with a brigade of reindeer herders. Living among wolves amid the snow blizzards and sub-zero temperatures, the herders' lives were packed with adventure and eustress, and as a result they could find health and happiness in some of the most hostile places on earth.

ARCTIC ADVENTURE: COLD, HARD TRUTHS

LOCATION: Olenyok, Siberia
PROJECT: Apprentice Reindeer Herder
TEMPERATURE: −40°C

It's March 2008 and I am a (trainee) Evenki reindeer herder. Geographically, I'm in the Russian wilderness high above the Arctic Circle, but physically I am somewhere between frostbite and exhaustion. For the past five days we've travelled 145 miles across bleak, mountainous terrain called a tundra (specifically within Yakutia Siberia). Moving by foot, sled and snow our goal was simple: move eighty precious reindeer to new pastures and protect them within one of the world's most hostile environments.

Needless to say, my short, stubby legs and English physiology was struggling in the snow and sub-zero temperatures, but despite being entirely out of my depth I had complete faith in my hosts and mentors. This is because reindeer herding is more than a profession for the Evenki of Siberia: it forms the very core of their culture and has done so ever since the first reindeer was domesticated and saddled over 400 years ago. This allowed the Evenki to travel in teams (known as brigades) over previously impenetrable lands in temperatures as low as −40°C, which is why over the years they are estimated to have covered an area of seven million square kilometres in Eastern Siberia.

Working, travelling and living in conditions that would kill most within a matter of hours, this land of extremes offers little room for error, and things can change from dangerous to outright deadly within seconds. But the thing that continued to amaze me about my Evenki brothers was their nomadic way of life had remained relatively unchanged for centuries, and not only had they learned to survive out here, they'd also learned to thrive.

Happily trekking across some of earth's most treacherous terrain, my brigade brothers epitomised this idea I called *Healthy and Happy Hardship* by embracing eustress. In a single day, I'd witness them cover thirty miles by sled, undertake hours of back-breaking labour wrestling with their reindeer, only to then follow the day's activities with what they describe as an evening of 'BOOM! BOOM!' when their wives and girlfriends visited the camp.

What was the secret to their superhuman stamina, virility and ability to please their loved ones in temperatures that would ordinarily shrink and shrivel a man's 'vital' organs? Well, it seems a profound understanding of ancient philosophy and an age-old technique of 'half-castration'.

Yes, it's as odd as it sounds.

But it was only on my final day as an Evenki herder that I came to learn about all of the above. This is because on day six we reached our ultimate destination where the reindeer would stay throughout spring. At this rural and semi-derelict corral, one of our final tasks was to separate the males from the females into different pens. This job alone took five hours to move all eighty, since reindeer can weigh up to 200 kg and if they're not willing to move (which many weren't) you'd essentially have to push, pull and wrestle 200 kg of deadweight through seemingly endless, towering snowdrifts.

Thankfully, before the sun began to set, I managed to drag the last (and most reluctant) reindeer into its enclosure. Bruised and battered from being 'dry humped' by a herd of reindeer, I then walked over to the chief of our brigade for further instructions.

His name was Nikolai Mikhailovich. Standing 5 ft 5 in tall and 65 years old, like most Evenki he was deceptively strong for his small frame and had been utterly weathered by the Siberian wilderness, years and miles of wisdom visibly etched into the wrinkles on his face. Not speaking a word of English (and with my grasp of the Evenki language still woefully poor) we relied heavily on the translation skills of his right-hand man, Vadik. At 53, he'd also been visibly shaped by the snow and ice throughout the years, but had previous experience assisting American scientists researching climate change throughout the Arctic in the late 1990s. Being very intelligent, he then self-taught himself English so he'd be better equipped to lead foreigners through his homeland and now, years later, he was doing it again with an utterly clueless (yet highly keen) Englishman.

'What's next?' I asked exhausted.

Nikolai and Vadik conferred among themselves until deciding it was time I attempted to master another nomadic tradition that would both help the herd and combat climate change.

'Climate change is bad,' Vadik said, frowning and shaking his head.

'We must protect the reindeer,' he continued, pointing at his herd.

As an adventurer, I wholeheartedly agreed since I had witnessed its devastating effects all over the world, from the droughts in the Namibian desert with the Ju-Wasi San Bushmen to the deforestation of the Amazon in Brazil with the Yaminawá shaman.

'Yes,' I replied, eager to help.

'So, what can I do?'

His answer was one I was not expecting.

'You must now half-castrate the reindeer,' Vadik said.

I paused for a moment. Evenki practices were tried and tested over centuries. I wouldn't ever question their way of life, since it was clearly working. But I wondered how reindeer testicles would provide a solution to climate change. Nonetheless, I agreed to the request and asked for a knife as I awaited further instruction from Nikolai.

'No knife,' Vadik said sternly. 'We do it the traditional way, like our forefathers before us.'

Again, not wanting to question years of proud Evenki tradition, I asked if we'd be using spoons, forks or any other kitchen utensils.

'No, we use our teeth,' he replied, gesturing to his mouth as Nikolai nodded.

He then explained to me that years ago, the researchers he accompanied showed that (partially) sterilised male reindeers can grow larger in size so are better able to break through ice with their hooves to find the vegetation trapped beneath. But they are also more willing than the non-castrated males to forgo battles for territory and courtship during mating season and instead move aside and share food with calves that would otherwise die of starvation in bad winters.[2]

'Castrated reindeers help the survival of the entire herd,' Vadik said.

'Yes, but surely there's a better way than assaulting testicles with your teeth?' I ventured.

They then explained how using our teeth ensures the reindeer is only half-castrated. Essentially, you 'crunch' one testicle between your back (molar) teeth and then 'grind' it until it becomes 'mushy'. This means the reindeer is sterilised and more docile in nature but still has some testosterone coursing through its body to encourage muscle growth.

Moments later, a massive male reindeer with the largest testicles I've ever seen was laid on the floor and his legs spread apart and held down by members of the brigade. I then did what any polite Englishman would do in this situation. I leant down. Put the left testicle in my mouth. Positioned it between my back teeth. Then bit down.

What happened next is hard to describe, but there was a 'pop' followed by a 'crunch', which showed the procedure was working but not yet complete.

'Now grind down with your teeth,' Vadik instructed.

As soon as he said this, the reindeer (not surprisingly) began frantically kicking in protest at the strange man between his legs. Struggling to hold it down and unable to speak with a mouth filled with furry animal scrotum, I did as I was instructed. Now essentially chewing on a reindeer's sterilised testicle, I tried my best to complete the procedure as fast as possible (for both our sakes). Thirty seconds later, I emerged with a face covered in what was basically reindeer pubes and we watched as he ran back to his herd with his surgical procedure complete.

As a brigade, we then circulated our castration duties. Completing ten 'operations' in the corral that day before the sun went down, we took it in turns to either hold down the legs or be 'face down' (and teeth first) between the legs. But what continued to amaze me about the Evenki were the festivities that followed the final testicle chewing as my brigade brothers were reunited with their wives and girlfriends.

Taking shelter in a small, semi-permanent settlement of tents, I noticed that the structures themselves closely resembled the traditional tepees used by most nomadic hunter-gatherers. Held together by long poles, the conical-shaped architecture of each tent had a fireplace at its centre that provided warmth and a place to cook as the smoke was carried up and out of the gap in the roof.

Slumped into a comfortable mess by the fire, I was immediately surrounded by the brigade's children who found my beard somewhat of a novelty act, as most Evenki are cleanly shaven. Happy to provide the evening's entertainment, I then watched on as my brigade brethren celebrated long into the night with their loved ones, for a brutal but successful migration of the reindeer was now complete.

As I watched on, and more questionable bottles of what I think was vodka were served, I continued to be amazed by the Evenki's ability to find happiness in one of the world's most hostile environments. Kissing girlfriends and wives with mouths that were previously full of fuzzy reindeer genitalia and dancing with legs that had covered over 180 miles through mountainous snowdrifts, they truly understood *How to Adventure* and as a result had a profound and innate understanding of eustress and the long-lost concept of *eudaimonia*.

A term that originated in ancient Greece, eudaimonia was a word emphasised by renowned philosophers Plato and Aristotle and for me (and many others) it was a better word for 'happiness'. This is because today we're told the overriding rationale for our hobbies, work, relationships and the conduct of our daily lives is the pursuit of happiness. But ancient Greek philosophers believed this was too simplistic and the very term had many shortcomings.

By relying too heavily on the word 'happiness' we are frequently (and wrongly) programmed to avoid discomfort, fatigue, fear and testing situations.

This is why eudaimonia is better. Roughly translated as 'fulfilment', it's different from happiness since it openly accepts that pain and struggling should form part of the process. It's entirely possible to be fulfilled, but at the same time feel stressed and overburdened. This is a small yet significant psychological nuance that the word happiness doesn't address, since it is difficult to speak of being happy yet unhappy (or happy yet struggling) but it's why I believe we adventure.

Even in life, this is why Plato and Aristotle did not believe the purpose was to be happy – the purpose was to pursue eudaimonia. All because this word encourages us to trust that many of life's most worthwhile projects will come with a sizeable serving of suffering and struggle but are worth pursuing nevertheless. These could range from creating a new business, building your dream house or migrating reindeer 180 miles across some of the deadliest terrain Mother Nature has ever created.

Essentially, happiness without fulfilment is a failure.

This is why the ancient Greek philosopher Epictetus famously once said, 'The greater the difficulty, the more glory in surmounting it. Skilful pilots gain their reputation from storms and tempests.'

More than a thousand years later, on 10 April 1899, the great American President Theodore Roosevelt stated in his famous speech 'The Strenuous Life': 'I wish to preach, not the doctrine of ignoble ease, but the doctrine of the strenuous life, the life of toil and effort, of labour and strife; to preach that highest form of success which comes, not to the man who desires mere easy peace, but to the man who does not shrink from danger, from hardship, or from bitter toil, and who out of these wins the splendid ultimate triumph.'

This is fundamentally why witnessing a sunrise following a 20 km vertical hike up a mountain is so much more fulfilling than watching it on a screen from the comfort of your sofa. In the *Journal of Henry David Thoreau 1837–1861* the author, considered to be one of America's great modern philosophers, wrote about his daily practices one Christmas Day of 1856 when he said, 'Take long walks in stormy weather or through deep snows in the fields and woods, if you would keep your spirits up. Deal with brute nature. Be cold and hungry and weary.'

Days later in his diary he expanded on this point and wrote, 'We must go out and re-ally ourselves to Nature every day. We must make root, send out some little fibre at least, even every winter day.

I am sensible that I am imbibing health when I open my mouth to the wind. Staying in the house breeds a sort of insanity always.'

This is why we modern humans need adventure more than ever.

Not necessarily a large-scale expedition across miles, days, weeks or months, but rather an exciting experience that is typically a bold, sometimes risky, undertaking to avoid 'spiritual decay'. This term was inspired by the 1956 book *The Outsider* by Colin Wilson who wrote, 'A man has achieved his present position by being the most aggressive and enterprising creature on earth. And now he has created a comfortable civilisation he faces an unexpected problem . . . the comfortable life lowers a man's resistance so that he sinks into an unheroic sloth . . . the comfortable life causes spiritual decay just as soft sweet food causes tooth decay.'

Finally, this idea of suffering for success isn't just confined to the realms of philosophy. French-born, Nobel Prize-winning biologist Alexis Carrel believed that, 'To progress again, man must remake himself. And he cannot remake himself without suffering. For he is both the marble and the sculptor. In order to uncover his true visage, he must shatter his own substance with heavy blows of his hammer.'

In summary, it was the work of Plato, Aristotle, Roosevelt and Thoreau (along with my time with the Evenki in 2008) that taught me *Why We Adventure* to combat 'spiritual decay'. But it took me over a decade to combine their teachings and philosophies with sports science to produce a systematic, structured and scientific way to train for an expedition and to truly understand *How to Adventure*.

PART 2 |
HOW TO ADVENTURE

'There is no blueprint when attempting the impossible. You must create your own.'

Your physical fitness will greatly impact *How to Adventure*. For it's an unavoidable truth that without a certain level of strength, speed and stamina you will not be able to walk the Great Wall of China, catch waves on Bondi Beach in Sydney, raft the Grand Canyon in Arizona or trek to Machu Picchu in Peru.

To put it bluntly, if you're not fit enough certain adventures will be closed to you.

The good news is, the more physically fit you are the more attainable mountain peaks, ocean crossings and uncharted terrain become. When learning *How to Adventure* you must understand certain principles of sports science, which is exactly why I wrote this entire book (and specifically this chapter).

Now, obviously every adventure is different.

Each will require specific skills, personalised planning and individualised, intricate preparation. Therefore, it's not possible to write a 365-day programme for everyone, since it would be far too generalised; the Law of Biological Individuality (we're all more different than we are alike) means a training plan written for everyone is a training plan written for no-one.

By documenting my own training plan over 365 days, I will demonstrate how I was able to:

- Recover from the world's longest (1,780 miles) sea swim.
- Rebuild my body with the world's strongest man.

- Recalibrate my perception to pain with one of the world's greatest martial arts experts.
- Return to the sea to coach a swim many believe is impossible.
- Reassess my training to adjust to a global pandemic.

The reason I say 'recover' was because after 157 days at sea for the Great British Swim, my body was bruised, battered and plagued with fatigue. And the reason I say 'rebuild' was because in many ways I was starting from scratch when it came to my training, and my road to recovery was going to be plagued with doubts, fears and concerns that I wanted to document with 100 per cent transparency.

When people hear stories of great adventures, they so often only see the tip of the proverbial iceberg. Whether it's pictures of Edmund Hillary and Tenzing Norgay standing heroically on the 29,035 ft summit of Everest, or stories of Roald Amundsen pioneering our exploration of the South Pole. So often we're unaware of the hours of training, failures and injuries that had to happen for those expeditions to be successful.

This book aims to change that.

By documenting the hours (and miles) of training in between large-scale expeditions, it's my hope that through deconstructing my training you will be better able to see the 90 per cent of the iceberg that many people don't even know exists.

Why 365 days?

Because no single-workout, 7-day plan or 30-day guide (however good) is actually that meaningful. What truly matters is the cumulative effect of thousands of hours of training and learning that are scientifically and systematically programmed into a long-term plan that's applied and modified over time. We have known this since the ancient Greek Olympics when the philosopher Flavius Philostratus (170–245 CE) described how the greatest athletes of antiquity would plan their entire year's training down to the finest detail. Yet today, we're bombarded with promises of quick fixes and tips or (at best) mediocre plans that only extend to six weeks, but every single one is incomplete, inadequate and fails to consider the year in its entirety.

This book is different and takes the proven principle of periodisation and applies it to the great outdoors so you can increase your physical (and mental) capacity for a specific adventure.

ADVENTURE: 1 YEAR - MACROCYCLE

Periodisation has been used for thousands of years. Traditionally seen in elite-level sport, it's a method of managing an athlete's training through the year so that they 'peak' at the right time for a competition. According to the *Journal of Human Sport and Exercise*, periodisation is defined as the 'Methodical planning and structuring of training process that involve a systematic sequencing of multiple training variables (intensity, volume, frequency, recovery period and exercises) in an integrative fashion aimed to optimize specific performance outcomes at predetermined time points.'[1]

It sounds complicated but it's not.

From the early years of the ancient Olympics, athletes have followed a very simple but logical method of training. Sometimes training for up to 10 months before the Olympics, they would prepare, compete, relax, recover and repeat.[2] This is periodisation in its most basic form as the athlete follows training phases (now called Preparatory, Competitive and Transition phases).

First described by the Greek philosopher Flavius Philostratus, his books on athletic training were pioneering at the time and shaped strength and conditioning as we know it today, but much of his work has been destroyed by the passage of time.

Years later, the Russian professor Leonid Matveyev was the first to use the term periodisation to plan the phases of an athlete's training. Studying competitors from the 1952 and 1956 Olympics, he wanted to know why some achieved their personal bests while others didn't perform to their full potential. He then developed strategies for peaking at the right time, and as a result the concept of periodisation which Flavius Philostratus first developed was brought into the era of the modern Olympic Games.

Over the years, many periodisation paradigms[3] have been proposed across different sports,[4] with different athletes[5] of different ages.[6] But a common theme is the requirement to manipulate programme variables (such as training intensity and volume)[7] in order to improve performance, control fatigue and reduce the risk of injury.[8]

Worth noting is that periodisation is developed for professional athletes to 'peak' at specific events.[9] But this book is about taking elite-level principles and making them accessible to all who are willing to learn, so they are better able to tackle (and 'peak' for) a large-scale, physically demanding adventure of their own.

Yes, of course, some adventures require no training. But for the bigger and bolder expeditions that are wrapped in eudaimonia and eustress and require strength, speed and stamina, this book will explain how the *Periodisation of Adventure* can help.

So how does it work?

- Periodisation is (often) the division of a training year known as a **macrocycle**.
- This year-long plan (macrocycle) is divided into a series of smaller manageable phases known as mesocycles.
- Each **mesocycle** then targets a specific fitness component to improve (strength, speed, skill or stamina) and is often (logically) divided into autumn, winter, spring and summer.
- Every mesocycle is then further subdivided into microcycles which involve a number of training sessions appropriately interrelated in order to reach one or more specific objectives.
- It is generally accepted that a **microcycle** can range from a few days to 14 days in length[10] with the most common length being 7 days.

ADVENTURE: 4 SEASONS – MESOCYCLE

As a graph, your macrocycle (and mesocycles) looks like those on the following pages. Notice the macrocycle consists of all 52 weeks and offers a 'bird's eye' view of your year's training schedule. Also note the intensity and volume of training is strategically manipulated throughout the four mesocycles that follow the four natural seasons (winter, spring, summer and autumn) to allow the body (and mind) time to recover and adapt to training stress, ensuring you don't become fatigued and 'stale' from overtraining. Put simply:

- **Training intensity** refers to the level of effort a person exerts during exercise relative to his or her maximum effort.
- **Training volume** refers to the total amount of work that you perform whether that's running mileage, swimming distance or reps/sets during strength training.

As mentioned before, although this periodised plan is typically adopted by elite-level athletes, it is particularly useful when applying these sports science principles to adventure too. That's because by plotting your ability to adventure within the graph as well, you're able to see when you're optimally primed and ready to take on an expedition based on where you're at (physically) with your training and your ability to handle volume and intensity.

Interestingly, this method of changing your training with the changing of the seasons was partly inspired by ancient philosophy that believed the best plans were those that worked in harmony with nature. This is why the famous Roman Stoic philosopher and statesman known as Seneca (4 BCE–65 CE) once said, 'Let us keep to the way which Nature has mapped out for us, and let us not swerve therefrom. If we follow Nature, all is easy and unobstructed; but if we combat Nature, our life differs not a whit from that of men who row against the current.'

1. AUTUMN (RECOVER)

The focus is on 'active recovery' where both the volume and intensity of training is kept low, allowing the mind and body time to rest. Scheduling sleep is critical during this time, as well as understanding ancient and modern sports rehabilitation practices and the power of strength training and theories in evolutionary medicine to rebuild the durability of the joints, muscles and tendons.

2. WINTER (BASE)

The focus is to create an 'athletic base' with a high volume of training at a low intensity while also improving work capacity (the body's ability to perform and positively tolerate training of a given intensity or duration). This is achieved through a system of training called General Physical Preparedness (targeted at strength and endurance) that was pioneered in the old Soviet Union (1922–91), but is done under conditions that take inspiration from the Spartan warrior society of ancient Greece (431–404 CE) to build mental resilience as well as work capacity.

3. SPRING (BUILD)

The focus is on building on your 'athletic base' as the volume of training is kept high and the intensity of training is incrementally increased. At this point, training starts to replicate your chosen sport or adventure more closely as you train technique and specific energy systems based on the teachings of the Russian Conjugate

Sequence System of the 1960s and early 1970s and the Process of Achieving Sports Mastery. Put simply, this is a method, theory and philosophy of training that helps athletes specialise and refine their specific skills.

4. SUMMER (PEAK)

The focus is on 'peaking' as the volume of training is reduced but the intensity is increased. During this phase, training should really begin to replicate competition while at the same time ensuring that you are recovering as hard as you train.

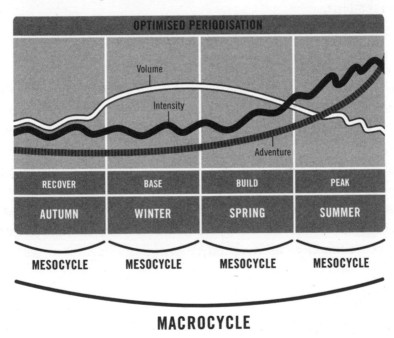

It's important to note here that if your event, expedition or adventure is in the winter then you must adjust your macrocycle (and order of mesocycles) accordingly. Since logic dictates that the winter period will be your peak mesocycle, if represented in a graph it would look like this (same concept, just a different order):

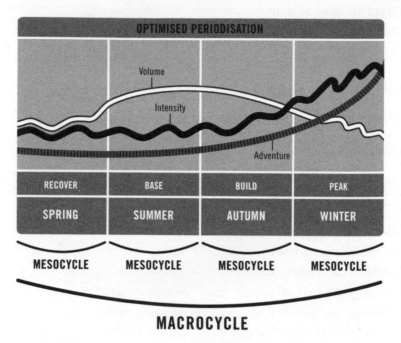

Finally, periodisation should not be considered a rigid programme to religiously follow. It's more a framework that we can (and should) adapt within. Too often, through strict reps, sets and regimes we're trying to apply a simple mechanical solution to a complex biological reality, but sports scientists now understand that a greater degree of flexibility is needed to work with our biological individuality.

To quote the *International Journal of Sports Physiology and Performance*, 'Such findings challenge the appropriateness of applying generic methodologies to the planning problems posed by inherently complex biological systems."[11] Basically, the body is a complex biological organism and thousands of variables impact on our training, recovery, nutrition and sleep. Therefore, in summary, don't be afraid to change your macrocycle, mesocycles and microcycles if you need to.

ADVENTURE: PLAN YOUR WEEK

MICROCYCLES

The smallest component of a periodised programme is known as a microcycle. Often lasting a week where the athlete focuses on a specific block of training, it's very important to maintain a balance between when your physiology should be placed under high stress and when that demand should be reduced slightly in order to allow for recovery, regrowth, regeneration and adaptation. At the most fundamental level, defining high, moderate and low intensity training days is a simple way to manage fatigue and ensure windows of recovery are available. An example of periodising a training week to get balance between the time an athlete is placed under high training stress and the time given to recovery may look like this:

Monday	Tuesday	Wednesday	Thursday	Friday	Saturday	Sunday
Moderate	High	Low	High	Low	Moderate	Off

This is particularly important during the first *Recovery Mesocycle* where adequate rest and recuperation *must* be considered during every training session.

ADVENTURE: DAILY HABITS

ASKESIS: HEALTHY HARDSHIP

'The comfort zone is the great enemy to creativity; moving beyond it necessitates intuition, which in turn configures new perspectives and conquers fears.'

Dan Stevens

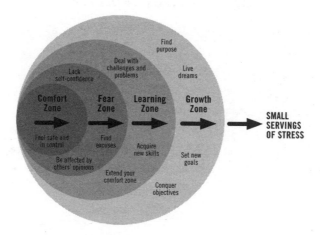

The term askēsis has changed over the years. It is now more commonly associated with 'asceticism' which is a lifestyle character-ised by abstinence from sensual pleasures often for the purpose of pursuing spiritual and religious goals. Its origins can be traced back to ancient Greece where the term *askēsis* originally meant 'training' or 'exercise' and didn't refer to self-denial but to the physical training required for athletic events. So when researching *How to Adventure*, I adopted this method of training that involves daily voluntary discomfort (and eustress) in nature to transform the mind and body. Examples of this include ice swimming, barefoot running and even forms of martial arts, where the focus isn't on the specific exercise but about practising a philosophy of healthy hardship.

BLUEPRINT: THE GOAL

Statistics show we humans are getting stronger, faster and fitter.

This is why every graph (in every sport) that plots the performance of Olympic athletes from 1896 (Athens) to 2016 (Rio) shows a steady rate of improvement.[12]

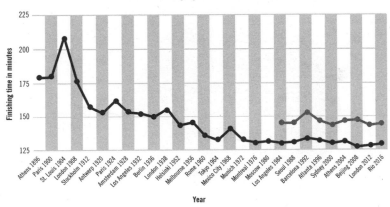

Gold medal winning times in the Men's and Women's marathon at the Summer Olympics from 1896 to 2016

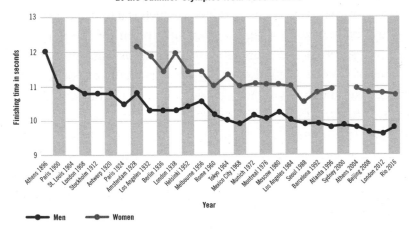

Gold medal winning times in the Men's and Women's 100 metre sprint at the Summer Olympics from 1896 to 2016

It's the same in the world of adventure too.

We're climbing faster, hiking further and venturing into ever more remote and hostile terrain that would have been considered impossible by great adventurers of old. Why? One reason is our understanding of sports science and application of tried and tested strength and conditioning principles. Over time this has allowed us to tweak and tailor our physiques and physiology so that each new generation of athlete is superior to the one before.

Marathon running

The highest level of marathon runner tends to have a low body-mass index (BMI) compared to other athletes. This helps with the biggest issue facing long distance runners: overheating. The shorter and slimmer a runner is, the larger surface area they have with which to dissipate heat. Over the last 50 years the average BMI of world record breakers has hardly changed, whereas it's greatly increased in the general population.[13]

Rowing

Record-breaking rowers are often taller than average and have been getting taller and taller since the early days of the modern Olympiad. Tall rowers are heavier which increases drag, but this is balanced by the increased stroke length. The longer your body, the longer your stroke, so each stroke propels a tall rower that little bit further forward than that of a shorter rower.

Weightlifting

Conversely, record-breaking weightlifters have shorter arms and legs which provide increased leverage. In fact, the shorter (and lighter) you are, the higher percentage of your body weight you can lift.

Sprinting

We are used to seeing Usain Bolt speed to victory in the 100m but he is much taller than the champion sprinters of the 20th century. Across the board, the centre of gravity of sprinters has risen, which helps in a number of ways; that high centre of gravity falls forward faster and more muscular arms help to counterbalance the power firing through the legs, helping with balance. However, the longer legs associated with height make it harder to accelerate.

Swimming

Being tall also helps you become a champion swimmer, as the water supports the extra weight. World record-breaking swimmers have been getting taller and faster over the last century. The ideal is a long torso, longer arms and shorter legs, as this helps with aerodynamics and power.[14]

Now, obviously all Olympians were born with a genetic predisposition to be suited to their chosen sport. Then – whether they were naturally tall, strong or fast – they were able to harness their genetic advantage with proven theories of sports science. This is why the *British Journal of Sports Medicine* states: 'That although deliberate training and other environmental factors are critical for elite performance, they cannot by themselves produce an elite athlete. Rather, individual performance thresholds are determined by our genetic make-up, and training can be defined as the process by which genetic potential is realised."[15]

In short, training is the realisation of one's genetic potential. Which is exactly why I decided to write this book. Since whatever your level of ability, age, weight or height, the information contained within these pages will equip you with the training principles you need to reach your 'genetic potential'. Which all begins with your Autumn Mesocycle.

AUTUMN | RECOVERY MESOCYCLE OVERVIEW

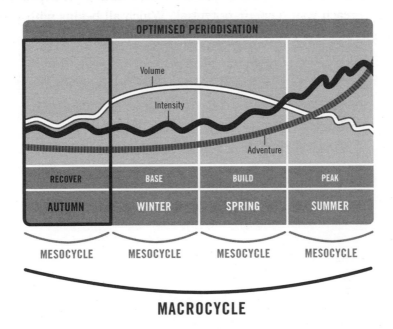

OPTIMISED PERIODISATION

Volume

Intensity

Adventure

| RECOVER | BASE | BUILD | PEAK |
| AUTUMN | WINTER | SPRING | SUMMER |

MESOCYCLE   MESOCYCLE   MESOCYCLE   MESOCYCLE

MACROCYCLE

'RECOVER AS HARD AS YOU TRAIN'

After any extreme event or expedition, you must prioritise a *Recovery Mesocycle*. This is why you will notice both the volume and intensity of training during this period is kept very low as the goal is to rehab from an athletic adventure, reset imbalances within the body (both biochemical and physiological) and restore the healthy function of your sympathetic and parasympathetic nervous system to fully rest and recover.

Let's take the sport of ultra-marathon running as an example and specifically the Western States Endurance Run, a 100 mile (161 km) ultra-marathon that takes place in California's Sierra Nevada Mountains each year over rugged mountain trails and in brutal conditions.[16] Runners ascend a cumulative total of 18,090 ft (5,500 m) and descend a total of 22,970 ft (7,000 m), but because of the sheer length and brutality of the course it starts at 5 a.m. and continues throughout the day and into the night. Runners finishing before the 30-hour time limit for the race receive a commemorative bronze belt buckle, while runners finishing in under 24 hours receive a silver belt buckle. After studying participants, researchers found:[17]

- 50 to 60 per cent of the participants experienced musculoskeletal problems.
- Creatine kinase levels were high in the blood (CK is an enzyme that measures muscle damage).
- There were significant changes in heart functionality as shown by changes in cardiac biomarkers measured through electrocardiography and echocardiography.
- Digestive problems and gastrointestinal bleeding were common.
- There was a reduction in renal function (regulating fluid balance and electrolytes within the body, clearing toxins and enabling the production of various hormones).
- There were increased incidences of upper respiratory infections (problems with the nose and throat).

Finally, researchers concluded there was overall dramatic changes to 'Biomarkers indicating a pathological process (an organic process occurring as a consequence of injury and stress) in organ systems such as skeletal muscles, heart, liver, kidney, immune and endocrine system.'

All things considered, the body has a lot to cope with.

Which is why at the end of 2018, following my 1,780 mile swim around Great Britain in 157 days, I had to begin my *Recovery Mesocycle* and my goals needed to become focused on:

- **Scheduling Sleep.** Based on numerous studies that detail the rejuvenating and recovery-boosting properties of sleep, I researched how to restore the healthy function of my sympathetic and parasympathetic nervous system to combat chronic fatigue.
- **Ancient and Modern Sports Rehab.** Founded on thousands of years of research (and evolutionary medicine), I would separately rebuild my upper body and lower body through tried and tested sports science theory and philosophy.
- **Restructure the Body with Strength Training**. I would begin to strengthen the muscles, ligaments and tendons once again with the scientific, strategic and systemic use of strength training using bodyweight exercises, barbells and resistance bands.

Which all started at the Wilmslow Hospital in southwest England, with an injury that threatened to end my career as an ultra-distance sea swimmer.

STARTING MY RECOVERY MESOCYCLE: UPPER BODY
AUTUMN 2018, WILMSLOW, ENGLAND

It's 14 November 2018 at the Wilmslow Hospital. More specifically, I find myself lying inside a giant MRI (magnetic resonance imaging) machine as doctors closely inspect my muscles, ligaments, tendons and organs to make sure they are all intact, healthy and still functioning. This is because I'd been back on land a total of 10 days since setting the record for the World's Longest Sea Swim and while stories in the media heralding the swim as 'heroic' were incredibly appreciated, the harsh reality was no human had ever spent 157 days swimming 1,780 miles at sea and as a result there were bound to be consequences to my health.

Deep down I think I knew this, I just didn't want to admit it to myself. But the truth is my body (especially my shoulders) had begun creaking, cracking and complaining more than usual and it felt like I'd aged 20 years during my time at sea. Research published in the *Journal of Human Sport and Exercise* which analysed the age of peak performance in athletes would back that up.[18] According to scientists, at the London 2012 Olympic Games, '72% of the athletes were aged between 20 and 30 years [the average age for men was 26.2 and for women at 25.2].'

At 33 years old, I was obviously the wrong side of this statistic. This meant I had to make peace with the fact I was no longer the same athlete who ran a marathon (26.2 miles) while pulling a 1.4 tonne car, climbed a rope the height of Everest (8,848 m) and did a triathlon carrying a 100 lb tree injury free . . . in a single calendar year . . . without any physiotherapy or professional help.

But that's ok, I wasn't upset about it. Like all great older athletes, what I lacked in youth I was prepared to make up for in hard-earned experience and newly acquired knowledge, while financially investing in my body, especially after my body had been so kind to me. This was heavily inspired by an article I read about basketball legend LeBron James who reportedly spends $1.5 million a year on his body with cryotherapy, hyperbaric chambers, private chefs and more. As a result, many people believe that at 36 years old he's actually getting better with age and rewriting the rulebook on what an older athlete is capable of.

This explains why, in choosing to follow the 'LeBron Blueprint', I had recruited one of the UK's best shoulder experts, Professor Lennard Funk, to help fix my bruised and battered body. Waiting for me as I emerged from the MRI machine, this was his verdict.

'I'm amazed you were able to keep swimming,' he said.

'Oh, I know,' I replied. 'Usually the weather and waves around the British coastline are so unpredictable, but we got lucky and this season the sea was kind to us.'

'No, you don't understand,' he said, looking at the scan of my shoulder. 'You must have been swimming miles upon miles as the end of your clavicle [collarbone] was deteriorating and eroding away.'

'Oh,' I replied dumbfounded.

'Basically, this would have caused stress fractures along the end of the bone that are causing the creaking and cracking you're referring to. It would have been like swimming with a cheese grater in your shoulder,' he said, now visibly grimacing with empathy.

Pointing to the scan, he then told me it's an injury called Distal Clavicular Osteolysis that's caused by overuse, repetitive stress and trauma. Anatomically, the shoulder is made up of three bones: the scapula (shoulder blade), the humerus (upper arm bone) and the clavicle (collarbone). The acromioclavicular (AC) joint is where the end of the collarbone (closest to the shoulder) attaches to the acromion (a curved piece of bone that comes from the shoulder blade across the top of the shoulder). The clavicle and acromion meet to form the acromioclavicular joint in front of the shoulder. Ligaments and soft tissues then hold the acromioclavicular joint together and provide stability. But it's the repetitive trauma from training (or

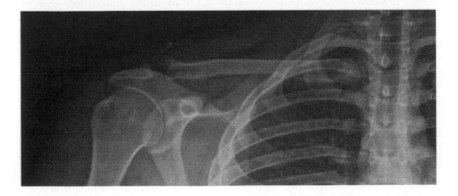

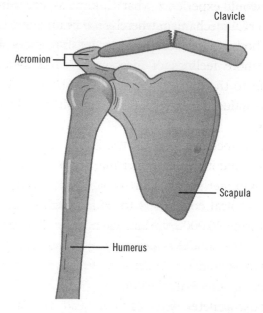

Clavicle

Acromion

Scapula

Humerus

in my case swimming) that causes tiny fractures of the distal end of the clavicle bone to produce Distal Clavicular Osteolysis.

'It must have been so painful,' he continued.

I nodded, but explained my shoulder was often the least of my concerns when swimming with a jellyfish tentacle hanging from my face was a daily occurrence.

'No, but did you not realise? Surely you could feel it?' he continued questioning me, confused as to why I was so oblivious to the bone grinding into my tendons and cartilage 12 hours a day, for 157 days.

I sat there for a moment in silence trying to think back to the swim, but the truth is I didn't realise. I was so tired, exhausted and preoccupied with outswimming storms that my entire body and brain was numb and refused to register pain and fatigue anymore. This is why in my book *The Art of Resilience* that documented the swim, I likened my state to that of an injured animal clinging to survival who would experience what's known as stress-induced analgesia,[19] a powerful mechanism whereby the brain alters the biochemistry in the body to release pain-suppressing endorphins so the animal can ignore feelings of discomfort[20] and instead fight for survival, often to the death if needed.[21] But now back on land any form of stress-induced analgesia had worn off, so I had to face the consequences.

Talking more specifically about the injury to the shoulder itself, Professor Funk said it wasn't surprising. Studies show, 'The average competitive swimmer swims approximately 60,000 to 80,000 m per week. With a typical count of 8 to 10 strokes per 25 m lap, each shoulder performs 30,000 rotations each week. This places tremendous stress on the shoulder girdle musculature and glenohumeral joint and is why shoulder pain is the most frequent musculoskeletal complaint among competitive swimmers.'[22] This is why most swimmers (and most athletes who play overhead motion sports) must give their shoulders some much needed tender, love and care during their *Recovery Mesocycle* to avoid common rotator cuff injuries (tendinopathy, rotator cuff tears, shoulder impingement, bursitis and labral tears).

Unfortunately, I wasn't like 'most swimmers'. I had swum 1,780 miles in waves and weather that contorted and tormented my rotator cuff, which is why that day I was faced with two options:

- Stop ultra-distance swimming (around countries), hang up the trunks and goggles and find a new sport, or
- Have surgery, pray it was a success and hope I could continue doing the sport that I loved and continue floating across oceans.

Now, if you understand the ancient Greek concept of eudaimonia, you will know why there was never any doubt that I was going to choose option 2. So I asked Professor Funk to book me into surgery

at his earliest convenience and cut whatever needed to be cut. All so
I could begin rebuilding my body, from the ground up, and return to
the sea as soon as possible.

REST AND REHAB, BUT REFUSE TO QUIT

It was 10 a.m. on 16 November 2018 when I awoke from surgery. A
very sweet, softly spoken nurse was there to tell me that they had
'shaved' the end of my clavicle and 'hoovered' out any loose bone
and debris that had broken off sometime during my swim and had
been floating around in my shoulder ever since. She then helped me
put on my trousers and sent me on my way with my arm in a sling
and a bag full of medicine as I practically skipped out the hospital,
high as a kite and unable to feel a thing, medicated on morphine and
painkillers.

Arriving back home, I took the afternoon off to recover but by the
evening was back training. Obviously, swimming, weight training
and anything that involved having two fully functioning shoulders
was out of the question, but a session sat on the bike with my arm in
a sling was allowed.

Now, it almost goes without saying that this wouldn't go down
as the greatest training session I'd ever completed. No personal
bests were broken and the wattage on the bike was woefully
low, which led me to believe the cocktail of opiates I'd been given
were not performance enhancing in any way. But that's ok, since
this session was more of a mental victory than anything. It represented (to myself) a sheer refusal to quit in the face of adversity,
and for many injured athletes and adventurers that's just as
important.

Of course, I wasn't the first athlete in history to be injured while
trying to push the limits of human potential and I won't be the last.
Perhaps the best example of this comes in the form of the martial

arts icon Bruce Lee whose incredible conditioning routines were legendary. With a profound understanding of human movement and musculature, a staple of his strength training was the 'good morning' exercise which is particularly good for strengthening what's known as your posterior chain (put simply, the backside of the body). He understood that by making the lower back, glutes, hamstrings and calves as powerful as possible he would be able to run faster, jump higher and kick harder than ever before.

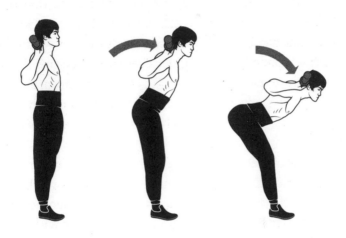

But on 13 August 1970, he was performing 'good mornings' with 60 kg (135 lb), his bodyweight at the time, when he heard a loud popping sound in his back. For several days, he tried heat treatments and massage, until the steadily increasing pain forced him to seek medical advice. Now it's unclear whether it was the volume or intensity of training that caused the injury (potentially both) but it's believed he had severely damaged his sacral nerve (located in the sacral plexus in his spine) which is needed for the efficient function and movement of the posterior chain, lower leg and foot. After assessing the severity of the condition, doctors told him he would no longer be able to train in martial arts ever again and may even struggle to walk.

Understandably devastated by the news, Bruce was then ordered to remain in bed for six months while he recovered. But it wasn't in his nature to lay there and do nothing. No, during this time he began studying the human body, his injury and the best methods of rehab and recovery. Essentially, researching and writing his own *Blueprint* to rebuild his bulletproof body, Bruce Lee became a true pioneer of sports science and began cross-pollinating ideas from anywhere and everywhere. His reading list included:

- *On Fencing* by Aldo Nadi.
- *Aikido: The Arts of Self-Defense* by Koichi Tohei.
- *Aikido* by Kisshomaru Ueshiba.
- *Advanced Karate* by Mas Oyama.
- *A Beginner's Book of Gymnastics* by Barry Johnson.
- *Championship Fighting* by Jack Dempsey.
- *Book of Boxing and Bodybuilding* by Rocky Marciano.
- *How to Box* by Joe Louis.
- *US Army Boxing Manual.*
- *Efficiency of Human Movement* by Marion Ruth Broer.
- *Physiology of Exercise* by Laurence Morehouse.
- *Wing Chun Kung-Fu* by James Lee.
- *Acupuncture: The Ancient Chinese Art of Healing* by Felix Mann.
- *Esquire's The Art of Keeping Fit.*
- *Combat Training of the Individual Soldier* by the US Army.
- *Modern Bodybuilding* by Oscar Heidenstam.
- *The Athlete in the Making* by Jesse Feiring Williams and Eugene White Nixon.
- *Bodybuilding: The Official Training Textbook of the British Amateur Weightlifting Association* by John Barrs.
- *Dynamic Judo: Throwing Techniques* by Kazuzo Kudo.
- *Dynamic Judo: Grappling Techniques* by Kazuzo Kudo.
- *Dynamic Self-Defense* by Sam H Alred.

This is just a small sample of his strength and conditioning library and doesn't even list his books on Eastern and Western philosophy. But what it does demonstrate is his sheer refusal to quit and his resolute will to recover, even in the face of adversity and professional medical advice. Did it work? Well, although it was reported he suffered chronic back pain for the remainder of his life, he found a way to resume his martial arts training and starred in four (and a half) films made between 1971 and 1973. All while he continued to teach his martial art of Jeet Kune Do to the world.

ROAD TO RECOVERY

A few weeks passed and my shoulder, although still weak, was free from the sling and I was given the 'green light' to begin physiotherapy, rehab and shoulder-strengthening exercises.

Upon hearing the news, I immediately enlisted the help of my long-time friend and chief physiotherapist of all my ambitious swims, Jeff Ross. Renowned within the world of rehab, he was usually tasked with caring for the physiology of elite athletes ranging from New Zealand's Rugby League team to Premier League footballers here in Britain. But somehow our paths crossed and now his clinic in Wilmslow was frequently visited by me as I invested in my body and followed the 'LeBron/Lee Blueprint'.

'So, what range of motion are we working with?' Jeff asked.

"Hmm . . . pretty bad,' I replied. 'Basically, I can just about drink a cup of tea, but brushing my hair or wiping my bum is currently considered too mobile for me.'

Jeff began laughing, but was completely unfazed. He'd treated me in a urine-soaked wetsuit with seaweed stuck in my beard before, so there were very few personal boundaries left between us.

'What about strength?' he asked.

'Honestly, I'd struggle to bench two kilos right now,' I admitted, not knowing what hurt more, my ego or shoulder.

'That's ok. This is a chance to recover and reprogramme your training. We're going to rebuild you. Like Bruce Lee in *Enter the Dragon*, making you even stronger and even more durable than before . . . like Ross 2.0.'

I smiled, since I did love the reference.

He then explained that often rehab is a fine line between recovering and gradually, slowly and progressively building back strength.[23] This is because strength underpins everything we do and it is the accumulation of strength over a period of time that allows all of our body's structures to adapt and make us less prone to injury. This principle applies to bones, muscles, joints, ligaments or tendons: all of them have the ability to adapt to the forces that are placed upon them. If we load too quickly we get injured (or re-injured), since we have not accustomed the body and its structures to that weight, volume or intensity. On the other hand, if we increase the load gradually, our body and its structures adapt and we become stronger and more resilient.[24]

For those interested in the science, what Jeff was referring to here was what's known as *Mechanotransduction*. According to the *British Journal of Sports Science*[25] this is, 'The physiological process where cells sense and respond to mechanical loads (weight and force)' and explains how, 'Load (weight and force) may be used therapeutically to stimulate tissue repair and remodelling in tendon, muscle, cartilage and bone.'[26]

It sounds complicated, but it's not. In fact, the body is in a constant state of flux with its physical and connective tissues, responding to the world around us to maintain optimal levels of connective tissue required for activity. We respond to load and stimulus, and this makes our body continually adapt and re-model all the time.[27] This is where the term *mechanotherapy* comes from. This is, 'The employment of mechanotransduction for the stimulation of tissue repair and remodelling.' Put simply, it is the use of load and mechanical stress to help us heal, repair and strengthen. This is why rest and recovery is so important during any *Recovery Mesocycle*, but that's not to say you shouldn't do anything at all and get lazy. On the contrary, a well-structured programme (rooted in mechanotherapy) could be the key to transforming an injured, frail or fatigued musculoskeletal system from sick to strong.

FROM SICK TO STRONG

The goal of every *Recovery Mesocycle* is to rehab and recover while at the same time re-build strength. The sports science genius Tudor O Bompa agrees too. Recognised worldwide as the foremost modern expert on periodisation training, he first developed the concept of 'periodisation of strength' in Romania in 1963, as he helped the Eastern Bloc countries rise to dominance in the athletic world. He stated, 'Whether parallel with the rehabilitation of injuries, or afterwards, before this phase ends all the athletes should follow a program to strengthen the stabilisers, the muscles which through a static contraction secures a limb against the pull of the contracting muscles. Neglecting the development of stabilisers, whether during the early development of an athlete or during his peak years of activity, means to have an injury prone individual, whose level of maximum strength and muscular endurance could be inhibited by weak stabilisers. Therefore, the time invested on strengthening these important muscles means a higher probability of having injury free athletes for the next season.'[28]

This is supported by the *British Journal of Sports Medicine* which stated that, 'Strength training reduced sports injuries',[29] following their research to determine which training protocol (strength training, stretching or proprioception conditioning) was most effective at reducing sports injuries.

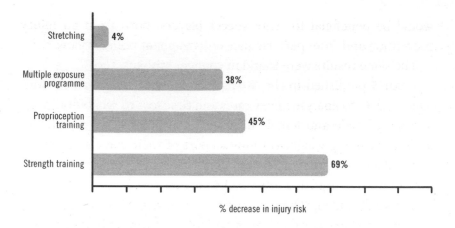

% decrease in injury risk

After studying 26,610 participants with 3,464 injuries what they found was, 'Strength training reduced sports injuries to less than 1/3 and overuse injuries could be almost halved' and performed better than both stretching or proprioception conditioning routines.

Led by the same chief researcher (and again published in the *British Journal of Sports Medicine*) they also found this to be true in studies around the world, 'despite considerable differences in populations'. They found, after analysing 7,738 participants aged 12–40 years in studies published in 2003–2016, that, 'Increasing strength training volume and intensity were associated with sports injury risk reduction.'[30]

The same results were found in elite athletes. Research from the *Scandinavian Journal of Medicine and Science in Sports* wanted to, 'Evaluate whether a preseason strength training programme for the hamstring muscle group could affect the occurrence and severity of hamstring injuries.' Sports scientists had soccer players perform a supplementary (extra) strength training session 1–2 times a week for 10 weeks by using a special device aiming at specific eccentric overloading of the hamstrings. Hamstring injuries were registered during the total observational period of 10 months.

The results showed injuries were vastly reduced and, 'That addition of specific preseason strength training for the hamstrings would be beneficial for elite soccer players, both from an injury prevention and from performance enhancement point of view.'[31]

The same results were found in younger athletes, too.

A study published in the *Strength and Conditioning Journal* was, 'Undertaken to analyse injury rates and time lost to rehabilitation in a group of male and female high school athletes (ages 13–19). All athletes utilizing weight training as part of their exercise program suffered an injury rate of 26.2 per cent while their counterparts who did not were injured at a rate of 72.4 per cent.'

The study added, 'The rehabilitation ratio (time lost to rehabilitation due to injury per number of athletes performing in the studied group) was 4.82 days for control group athletes vs. 2.02 days in athletes who trained with variable resistance exercise.'[32]

Guess what? The same results were found in older athletes, as well.

A review published in the *Scandinavian Journal of Medicine and Science in Sports* aimed to analyse, 'The role of exercise in the reduction of risk factors and the prevention of falls and injuries' in elderly subjects caused by, 'Low strength and power, poor balance, poor gait and functional ability.'

They concluded, 'This review highlights the necessity of tailored, specific balance and strength exercise in the multidisciplinary prevention of falls and injuries.'[33]

These are just a handful of studies, but it shows on a large-scale across sports, countries, age groups and gender that strength training could hold the key to creating robust and resilient humans during a *Recovery Mesocycle*.

FORGE STRENGTH IN FORGOTTEN MUSCLES

Back in the clinic Jeff stressed that, 'It's also so important we build this strength in the right places. For the shoulder, this means conditioning the smaller, often forgotten muscles that stabilise and hold the scapula in a good position. If these are strong, we can "pile" load on top of that and the shoulder will cope. If they're not, the shoulder will continue to struggle.'

'Where can I find these *forgotten muscles*?' I asked.

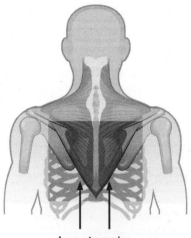

Lower trapezius

Jeff then proceeded to draw a series of diagrams on the giant whiteboard he keeps in his clinic while demonstrating movements on a life-sized skeleton as he explained how the lower trapezius plays a crucial role in 'ideal' scapula mechanics[34] and how poor scapula movement during overhead activities may mean the athlete is predisposed to injury in the form of impingement, subacromial bursitis and instability.[35]

He then said, 'Don't worry about the technical names, but see how the lower trapezius work to pull, push and rotate the scapula which then allows the arms to operate over a large range of motion?'

I nodded and was now weirdly conscious of my lower trapezius and scapula.

Jeff continued, 'Think of your lower trapezius and scapula like the roots and trunk of a tree and the large branches attached to this as your arms. If the foundations and base of the tree is unstable, weak or broken in anyway the branches will also feel unstable, weak and broken. But if it's strong, every other movement becomes strong, from your heaviest overhead press to your fastest tennis serve and your top swimming speed.'

Needless to say, I was sold on the shoulder science and immediately wanted the strongest lower trapezius in the Seven Seas, which is why Jeff then explained why resistance bands would be the best tool I have in my strength and condition arsenal and detailed more, tiny, forgotten muscles that are essential to creating a bulletproof body.

SHOULDER SCIENCE TO BUILD STRENGTH: RESISTANCE BANDS

The shoulder provides us with almost 360-degree movement in multiple directions. This is why we must also learn to comprehensively train the muscles and ligaments around the ball and socket joint in its entirety. To do this, we must strengthen the muscles of the rotator cuff which is where the resistance provided by bands can be invaluable.

Resistance bands are just elastic bands that can be used to add resistance to movements. But unlike barbells and our own bodyweight, they don't rely on gravity to provide resistance (like when hanging/brachiating) and can instead be worked over different ranges of motion. For athletes, this is particularly important since they allow them to train certain movements, under resistance, over more functional ranges of motion that better mimic those experienced during sport-specific activities.

Illustrating the importance of sport-specific ranges of motion, a study published in a 1998 issue of the *American Journal of Sports Medicine* reported a significant improvement in the shoulder strength and speed of serve in collegiate tennis players who trained using elastic bands.[36]

As you can imagine, trying to replicate that same action and resistance with a dumbbell alone would be quite hard if not impossible and certainly wouldn't yield the same results.

Furthermore, researchers from Louisiana State University found a resistance band training programme strengthened the rotator cuff muscles of baseball pitchers better than a barbell-based regime. Again, a resistance band would be far better at mimicking that range of motion compared to lifting dumbbells or throwing weighted medicine balls around the weights room.[37]

Put simply, this is all because free weights can only really apply resistance in a vertical plane, thanks to gravity. But resistance bands help you operate over a horizontal plane that could better replicate swinging a racket or the throwing of a ball and are better suited to training the rotator cuff, which is made up of four muscles. These work together to provide stability to the shoulder and keep the joint in the best position. All four muscles are attached to the scapula (shoulder blade) and extend towards the humerus (upper arm) but each attach to a specific point on the humerus.

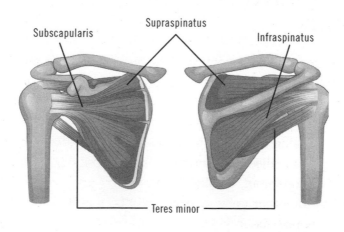

Anterior view   **Posterior view**

- **SUPRASPINATUS.** Located at top of the scapula. This muscle allows the shoulder to abduct or raise the arm and moves it away from the body.
- **SUBSCAPULARIS.** Found at the front side of the scapula, or when looking from behind it is tucked underneath the scapula. It allows the shoulder to internally rotate or turn the upper arm towards the body.
- **INFRASPINATUS & TERES MINOR.** Sit on the back of the scapula. They enable the upper arm to externally rotate or turn outwards away from the body. Although each rotator cuff muscle moves the shoulder in a specific direction, they work together to ensure that it is centred in the joint throughout all ranges of movement.

It's important to keep the ball of the humerus centred in the socket and the rotator cuff plays a significant role in doing so. If it is not, abnormal stress is placed on the surrounding tissue and cartilage which will make the shoulder susceptible to injury.

SHOULDER SCIENCE TO BUILD STRENGTH: BODYWEIGHT

Weeks passed and as I continued to build the small muscles in pursuit of Ross 2.0, I found the strength and range of motion of my shoulder was starting to return to its former glory. As a result, I was able to begin one of the simplest (but often neglected) forms of rehab . . . hanging. It sounds so simple, but when studying human evolution[38] you realise we humans are considered part of the great ape family (orangutan, gorilla, chimpanzee[39] and bonobo[40]). But while all of the other great apes can still be found swinging from trees, we stopped about 30,000 years ago. Fast forward to modern man and, despite sharing a similar shoulder structure, our joints aren't getting the exercise that nature intended and so they can weaken and become prone to injury.

This is why renowned orthopaedic surgeon John M Kirsch believes the simple act of hanging from a bar for up to 30 seconds, three times per day, can fix up to 99 per cent of shoulder pain. Outlining this protocol in his book *Shoulder Pain? The Solution and Prevention*, he believes the reason it works is because it brings back a long-lost form of shoulder prehab and rehab used by our evolutionary ancestors known as brachiating.[41]

Its name comes from the fact that it stretches the brachial artery, which supplies blood and nutrients to the arms, but aside from stretching the brachial arteries, the hang also stretches and strengthens the supraspinatus tendon. This is the tendon that's mainly responsible for shoulder strength, mobility and endurance.

When you raise your arms forward, the supraspinatus tendon gets pinched between your shoulder bones. That's where the pinching sensation comes from when you try to raise an injured or compromised shoulder. But when the arms are raised straight up as in the brachial hang, this gives the tendon room to move and stretch without getting pinched. This allows you to exercise, stretch and reshape this tendon and the surrounding muscles and bones. In short, the more you do the brachial hang, the better, stronger and more resilient your shoulders will be.

How do I know? Because just eight weeks after emerging from hospital, highly medicated with my arm in a sling, I was now back swimming and strength training thanks to the genius of Jeff Ross and Professor Lennard Funk. This is also why all the upper-body strength sessions detailed in this book begin with a series of bodyweight exercises and resistance band conditioning that I had tried, tested and lived by, all to ensure my shoulder joint was strong and bulletproof, all before any heavier weights were lifted.

STARTING MY RECOVERY MESOCYCLE: LOWER BODY
AUTUMN 2018, LONDON, ENGLAND

It's 10 a.m. on 7 December 2018 in Marylebone, London. It had been three weeks since my surgery, but now my shoulder wasn't my only problem. My legs and feet were complaining too. This is because during 157 days at sea I had barely used them (essentially skipping leg days for half the year), but now back on land and with an injured shoulder, all I could do was run, walk and bike. As a result, the muscles and joints in my lower body weren't too happy they were suddenly being asked to work so hard, which is why today I found myself *slowly* making my way towards the BXR clinic and training facility to have my sore, dishevelled sea body further analysed by Jeff and more experts. All to see why my legs and feet hated me and why I was incapable of running more than 5 km without feeling like something was going to snap, break or pop.

This is why during my walk there I emphasise the word 'slowly', since I had only been back on land a month and my 'sea legs' were still trying to remember what solid ground felt like. This explains why step after step my calves fatigued and tendons complained and why tube stations like Hampstead (London's deepest underground with 320 steps) would be considered suicide for my fragile feet.

Thankfully, I navigated the cobbled streets and by 10.30 p.m. was sitting in the waiting room exhausted. Collapsing into a seat, I rubbed my sore and suffering knees that were wondering what had just happened. As I did, I heard a softly spoken voice from across the room.

'Oh, my knees do that in the winter too.'

I looked up to see a sweet elderly lady, maybe 60 years old, with immaculately combed silver hair and a long, thick winter coat. I thought about telling her about the swim but didn't; she seemed so keen to help with her proposed remedies and I didn't want to interrupt her.

'Do you know what helps?' she said smiling, keen to share her wisdom.

'No, please do tell,' I said.

'A good pair of woollen pantyhose to keep those joints warm and supple,' she replied with a nod and smile, making her unsolicited advice all that much sweeter and appreciated.

About 30 minutes passed and I spent my remaining time in the waiting area hearing about the thermal properties of pantyhose. Turns out there's a lot I didn't know and they come in all sorts of colours and designs.

But by 11 a.m. it was clear I needed more than pantyhose to treat the many ailments that I'd collected from the ocean, as a team of experts gave their diagnosis on the damage caused to my shrivelled sea-swimming body. Starting with a diagnosis from Jeff, my morning went from bad to worse.

'Wow! That is quite remarkable,' he said as he examined my legs.

'I've never seen anything quite like it before,' he continued, but now searching for something on his laptop while taking notes.

'Oh really . . . good?' I foolishly asked.

'Oh sorry, no. Bad. In fact, terrible. I shouldn't have sounded so excited. It's just I've only ever read about severe muscular atrophy [degeneration of muscle function[42]] like this in astronauts who spend days and weeks in a weightless environment.'[43]

He then turned his laptop around to reveal research from NASA showing that, 'Prolonged exposure of human subjects to microgravity environment causes significant muscle atrophy accompanied by reduced muscle strength and fatigue resistance.'[44]

'You're like an astronaut returning from space,' he continued. 'Because you were swimming for 12 hours a day and suspended in water for 157 days, the muscles, ligaments and tendons in your lower body have shrivelled up and wasted away at sea.'

'Does this explain why my feet have turned all squishy and soft?' I asked.

'Yes, exactly – you're 33 years old with the feet of a newborn baby,' Jeff said.

I paused to consider his diagnosis. It made sense. In sports science, this is known as the SAID principle. Don't be fooled by the impressive sounding acronym – it stands for 'Specific Adaptation to Imposed Demands' and it just means you adapt specifically to the demands you place on your body.

This explains why tennis players[45] have a higher muscle mass and bone density in their dominant playing arm,[46] and why the *British Journal of Sports Medicine* states, 'Muscle imbalances exist in a wide range of athletes performing at the elite level and may be related to injury occurrence. Identification of the pattern of imbalance for different sports will enable muscle specific rehabilitation.'[47]

'How much atrophy[48] and muscle wastage are we talking?'[49] I asked.

'Well, the same study concluded, "Nine days of space flight may cause significant decreases in cross-sectoral areas [size] of the leg muscles," so not great,' Jeff said as he continued searching sports and medical journals for more answers.

'But to give an exact figure . . .,' he continued, 'research from the Maastricht University Medical Centre [Netherlands] calculated the rate of muscle atrophy from disuse [10–42 days] is approximately 0.5 to 0.6 per cent of total muscle mass per day although there is considerable variation between people.'[50]

Even without a calculator to run the maths it was clear my shrunken, squishy feet were not in the best shape after 157 days at sea and were in desperate need of some tender loving and care. Which is why looking at my macrocycle, it was clear I had to focus on the *Recover* (autumn) mesocycle which emphasises rest, rehab and re-acquiring strength and long-lost skills. It's essentially the exact same science that governed the rehabilitation of my shoulder, since according to thousands of studies (and coaching practices from many different sports) every properly periodised programme should not only focus on performance but also on an athlete's recovery and injury prevention.[51] This is especially important during this 'transition phase' (where an athlete finishes one macrocycle and prepares to start another) since the focus should be to restore injured muscles,[52] tendons, muscle attachments and joints through active rest, to remove the fatigue and replenish the exhausted energies.[53]

Of course, for my shoulder I already had a strength and conditioning routine and recovery protocol in place, but now I needed one for my lower body. 'Drilling down' into the detail, let's begin by understanding how the human body has successfully functioned for over 2.5 million years and why deviating too much from its original design could be a bad idea for modern man.

ANCIENT/MODERN REHAB

'When one's feet hurt, one hurts all over.'

This was a quote from the famous Greek philosopher Socrates. Although thousands of years old, modern sports science shows that it still holds true today. It was somewhat worrying for my squishy 'sea feet', since if left untreated research shows poor foot health can lead to the collapse of foot arches (or flat feet), arthritis or even stress fractures. Needless to say, I didn't want any of the above, which is why I found myself locked in the library at Vivobarefoot HQ with sleeves rolled up, elbows anchored deep in research. Delving into thousands of medical sports journals and owing much to the genius of Professor Dan Lieberman (Chair of the Department of Human Evolutionary Biology at Harvard) and Dr Peter Francis (Senior Lecturer in the School of Clinical and Applied Sciences at Leeds Beckett University) this is what I found.

Right now, there is a debate raging. It involves large, multi-million-pound shoe manufacturers and barefoot running advocates as both argue over the cause and cure for running-related injuries. Both agree that between 30 to 70 per cent[54] of runners incur running-related repetitive stress injuries[55] per year,[56] but they cannot agree on how to prevent, treat or cure these injuries. This is despite many perceived advancements in sports science and shoe technology in recent years.

There are many theories around this and right now there is no agreed scientific consensus on the correct one (I believe it's a blend of a few which I'll explain later). On the one hand, many believe running is just intrinsically 'harsh' on the body and bones and that high rates of injury are just normal (basically, the issue lies in the fragility of the human foot). Another widespread hypothesis is that many injuries result from 'training errors' when people run too far or too fast without properly adapting their musculoskeletal system (what this means is the issue lies in training methodology).

But it seems there's another emerging school of thought from the field of evolutionary medicine that looks to our ancestors for answers.[57] The basic idea behind this theory is that the human body survived and thrived and was moulded and adapted over millions of generations to cope with conditions during the Stone Age (8700–2000 BCE). But because farming and agriculture was invented less than 10,000 years ago (when we stopped being hunter-gatherers) it meant we humans rapidly changed our diets and environments, yet our biology remained the same. What this means is, our caveman (Palaeolithic) physiology cannot live in harmony with the modern environmental conditions that we have created for ourselves.

This is why problems can occur in both our food and our feet.

Addressing the former first, many nutritional scientists believe our ancestors were 'wired' to crave formerly rare nutrients like fat and sugar since both would provide valuable calories and energy during a dry season or famine. Basically, these cravings were key to our survival when we lived in a world where fats, carbs and calories were rare and hard to find. The problem is today we've developed cheap and plentiful supplies of calorie-dense foods and have cupboards and fridges stocked full of them. What this means is our primitive, caveman (Palaeolithic) brains and biology find it hard to function in an environment where we have a seemingly limitless supply of sweet, sugary calorific foods and also have to worry less about hunting, farming and famine. All things considered, from an evolutionary perspective, this 'mismatch' could help to explain the obesity epidemic.

LOW-INTENSITY STEADY STATE TRAINING AND ANCIENT/MODERN REHAB

But the logic of the 'mismatch hypothesis' can also be applied to our feet. As we know, the structure and function of the human foot and body has remained relatively unchained for millions of years. Therefore, in this context, we have been barefoot for almost the entirety of our existence (with the mass-market cushioned running shoe only arriving in the 1970s[58]) and seem to have done just fine. Yet today we wear big, padded shoes which from an evolutionary perspective is in conflict with nature, our caveman (Palaeolithic) physiology and the architecture of our feet and could (within the evolutionary medical hypothesis) be a cause or contributing factor to the deteriorating health of our feet.[59]

Why? Because it's believed modern shoes interfere with our natural running style, and since bad running technique is proven to make us more prone to injury, it makes sense that a more natural running style (to which the human body must have been adapted over millions of years) would help athletes avoid injury.

How? Through three inbuilt, primitive systems that overlap and interact when we run barefoot and come in contact with the ground. My issue (as will be the case for many reading this) was I had unlearned these three systems and if I attempted to run more than 10 km there was a risk that I too could join the growing number of injured athletes. Which is why I (and many others) must revisit, relearn and rehearse how to run properly, starting with:

1. BIOTENSEGRITY

The term 'biotensegrity' describes how all human tissue deforms and subsequently reforms. Everything from our heart, skin, muscles and tendons have been designed to behave in this way. In its most basic form, take your finger and press it against the skin on your arm and watch it deform and then reform when you let go. This is biotensegrity in action and the same happens when your foot strikes the floor.

Made up of 26 bones and 33 joints and supported by a complex mesh of ligaments, tendons and intrinsic foot muscles,[60] the architecture of our feet is very different to other primates, as the arches in our feet are capable of both stiffness[61] and deformation which helps us store and release energy via springs (ligaments, aponeurosis, tendons) in order to make efficient use of muscle work during running.[62] In fact, it is for this reason that the Achilles tendon is 10 times longer in humans compared with other primates,[63] as it serves as a 'spring' to propel us forward when running (when used correctly and like nature intended). Which leads us onto the second inbuilt, primitive system of the foot: sensory feedback.

2. SENSORY FEEDBACK

The human feet contain thousands of receptors that provide sensory feedback to the spinal cord for fast (reflex) responses and to the brain for overall control of movement. This is what's known as proprioception (also referred to as kinaesthesia) which is the body's ability to sense its own location, movements and actions and is the reason we're able to move freely without consciously thinking about our environment (like walking or running without looking at your feet).

For barefoot runners, proprioception is your best friend. Helpfully, it informs you if the terrain you're on is rough or smooth, flat or steep, stable or unstable. It even informs you how fast (or slow) you're running. All of which is invaluable when wanting to run with correct form to avoid injury, since this feedback allows us to tread lightly and avoid running-related repetitive stress injuries. The problem is that as soon as we wear shoes (and cover the soles of our feet) we lose the vital sense of proprioception and 'switch off' this sensory feedback. This in turn makes us 'numb' to our running technique as we no longer tread so lightly and become more prone to running-related repetitive stress injuries.

This is all closely related to the three ways our feet can strike the ground when running:

- **Heel Strike.** Where the heel of the foot lands first.
- **Midfoot Strike.** Where the heel and ball of the foot land simultaneously.
- **Forefoot Strike.** Where the ball of the foot lands first.

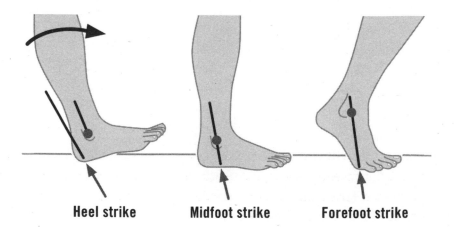

Heel strike   Midfoot strike   Forefoot strike

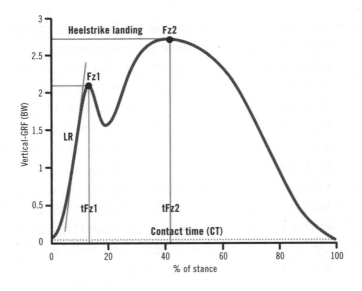

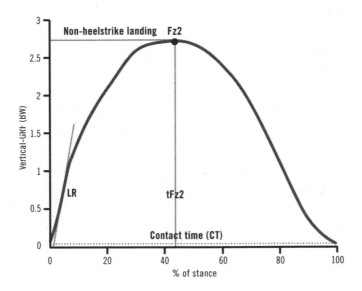

Often, we will use a variety of foot strikes depending on the terrain. But research shows our feet's inbuilt spring system works best when we use a midfoot or forefoot strike which allows the foot to stretch and recoil (biotensegrity) as the muscles move from eccentric (in tension but lengthening as our foot lands on the floor) to concentric work (in tension but shortening as our foot takes off from the floor).[64]

Now, it's believed humans ran with a mid to forefoot strike prior to the invention of running shoes.[65] But studies today claim an estimated 75 per cent of runners (recreational > 5 km) now use a heel strike[66] which has led some researchers to suggest that this is responsible for the increased risk of certain types of stress-related injuries[67] (like plantar fasciitis[68] and medial tibial stress syndrome[69]).

Why? Because different striking patterns exert different forces – and stress – on the body. If you look at the first graph where the runner's heel strikes, you'll notice an initial peak that shows the vertical ground reaction force. This is where a runner's foot lands on the outside of the heel and 'jabs' into the ground with a sudden impact.

Ouch! In this case the heel doesn't absorb any impact. It is just bone. This is more likely to occur in runners with cushioned shoes since that proprioception is 'switched off' and they may even be unaware they're heel-striking with so much force.

But runners who land on the forefoot – shown in the second graph – create relatively little impact force on the feet and that first peak of this graph where the heel was 'jabbed' into the ground is non-existent.

No ouch! In this scenario the ankle flexes and absorbs the impact. You're now using your ligaments, tendons, ankle and the foot's architecture like Mother Nature intended, and this is more likely in barefoot runners who have a greater degree of propriocep-tion and so understand the importance of managing ground reaction force.

This is supported by a study conducted at Harvard University in 2012 which said, 'Competitive cross-country runners incur high injury rates, but runners who habitually heel strike have significantly higher rates of repetitive stress injury than those who mostly forefoot strike.'[70]

Which leads us onto the third inbuilt, primitive system of the foot: our kinetic chain.

3. KINETIC CHAIN

The concept of the kinetic chain originally came from the German mechanical engineer Franz Reuleaux (1829–1905) when analysing how machinery works. He proposed that rigid, overlapping segments were connected via joints and this created a system whereby movement at one joint produced or affected movement at another joint in the kinetic link. In 1955, Dr Arthur Steindler (a renowned orthopaedic surgeon) expanded upon the work of Reuleaux and applied his concept of the kinetic chain to the human body and exercise to describe how the muscles, joints, fascia and nerves coordinate to produce movement.

Years later and our understanding of biomechanics continued to advance as we analysed the different ways we humans walk, jog, skip and run. These movements came to be called 'human gaits' and are essentially the different ways in which we can move, either naturally or from specialised training. As we've discovered, one key variable in running gait analysis is how our feet strike the floor, but our muscles throughout our entire body also provide a means of absorbing energy on landing and the position of the joint (leg) determines how effectively a muscle can work. For example, to lift an object you bend your elbows, usually to 90 degrees, so that your biceps are at mid-length (the optimum for lifting). If your arms were fully extended you could not generate as much force and if they were fully flexed you could not pick up the object. The exact angle you use comes from what you can see in front of you (e.g. how far or near/high or low the object is in space) and what information you are receiving (initially from your hands and subsequently from your muscles). Running barefoot allows your feet to experience sensation like your hands. The combination of systems 1 and 2 can then provide very precise information for your brain to use to optimise joint (leg) positions via muscles.

Now, it must be noted that technique will of course vary from runner to runner based on an individual's height, weight, bone structure and muscle mass. Therefore, despite what many experts will claim, the idea of the perfect running form doesn't really exist. But there are certain movements that are considered good and some that are considered bad and could result in injuries.

GOOD RUNNING TECHNIQUE

Taken from the *British Medical Journal*, the figure below shows, 'Humans' innate impact-moderating mechanisms on variable terrain. As the foot makes contact with the pebble (inset) it causes deformation of the skin and underlying tissues [biotensegrity].'[71]

This alters the position of the foot and the location and stimulation of the mechanoreceptors. Rapid and subtle adjustments are made via reflex arcs arising from stimulation of sensory nerves and modulation at the spinal cord (sensory feedback).

Based on this information (feedback) and visual input (feedforward) the brain directs motor output of the major muscles. Landing with a degree of flexion at the hip, knee and ankle provides mechanical advantage for muscles (gluteal, hamstrings, quadriceps, triceps surae) to absorb energy (eccentric control of deceleration) and generate propulsion during extension (concentric phase). Positioning the foot in the forefoot position (inset) on landing allows the Achilles tendon and the medial longitudinal arch (assisted by

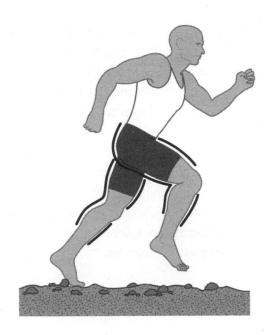
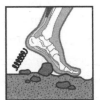

intrinsic foot muscles) to stretch as the heel comes towards the ground and rebound like a spring (kinetic chain).

BAD RUNNING TECHNIQUE

The proposed mechanism by which shoes may facilitate biomechanics which predispose some runners to certain types of injury. Cushioned footwear encourages a heel strike which is associated with an extended lower limb and a more upright torso. This in turn encourages a longer stride length in which the base of support is located further away from the centre of mass. In this position, the limb does not have mechanical advantage during ground contact which may encourage excessive breaking forces and increased repetitive tensile loading due to prolonged eccentric muscle contraction. One of the reasons these more 'blunt' running mechanics may occur is because

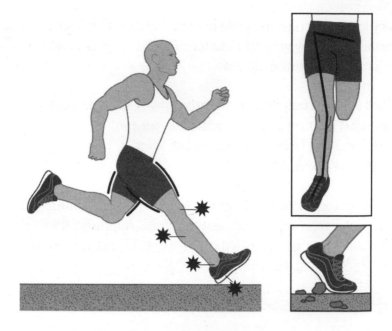

the foot (inset bottom) does not receive the same tissue deformation and sensory stimulation as it does in the barefoot condition.
Over time, this may lead to a reduced demand on posterior chain
muscles and a collapsing of the hip inwards in the frontal plane
(inset top). Running using these mechanics is perhaps also more
injurious because intrinsic foot muscles may be weaker from habitual footwear use (encouraging pronation, inset top) and lower limb
muscles (especially posterior chain) may be less conditioned from
modern sedentary lifestyles.

So, what does this all mean for my 'squishy sea feet'?

Well, Professor Dan Lieberman wrote in *Exercise and Sport
Sciences Reviews* that based on the evolutionary medical hypothesis
it's shown barefoot running can help encourage a more efficient
running technique. All because that's how the foot was designed to
function (biotensegrity, sensory feedback and an efficient kinetic
chain), which in turn can (logically) reduce our chances of injury.
Some runners may adopt this style naturally in shoes as they effort-

lessly forefoot strike and glide over the terrain with such grace and elegance that they generate less forceful impact peaks and stress on the joints. What this means is:

'How one runs may be more important than what is on one's feet, but what is on one's feet may affect how one runs.'
(Professor Dan Lieberman, Exercise and Sport
Sciences Reviews: April 2012)

All things considered, I think the Barefoot *v* Shoe running debate needs to be approached with less 'polarised thinking'. It's wrong to think shoes are good or evil, or that we should run barefoot or heavily cushioned. Instead:

- Be conscious about what you're putting on your feet (if anything).
- Understand how your choice of footwear (if any) impacts your running.

Ultimately, become a hybrid and use both.

Looking back through history, this was certainly true of the great East African runners. In his book *Barefoot Running Step by Step* the author Ken Bob says, 'It seems cliché to assume that every great East African runner grew up barefoot and trains barefoot, but a fact's a fact – that's what you see at the junior races at the cross-country championships in Kenya and Ethiopia. Young up-and-comers run them in bare feet because they have no other choice; they're unknown and have no shoe sponsor. As they mature, win internationally and attract sponsors they'll often run in shoes but maintain barefooting at home.'

A good example of this was Abebe Bikila of Ethiopia who won Olympic gold in the marathon in Rome in 1960, and Tokyo in 1964. But it was his performance in Rome that made the headlines. This was because Olympic sponsor Adidas were running low on shoes and didn't have a pair that fitted Bikila, but since he was already training in bare feet, he decided to run without shoes and took gold while quite literally showing the competition a 'clean pair of heels' as he crossed the finish line.

The same is also true of Eliud Kipchoge, a man who many considered to be the greatest marathon runner to have ever lived. For a member of the Nandi, the 'running tribe' of the high-elevation hills rising from the Rift Valley, the sweeping dirt roads would prove ideal barefoot training terrain and where the future champion could perfect his running style. Mile after mile, he drilled perfect technique (biotensegrity, sensory feedback and an efficient kinetic chain) until many years, medals and world records later he stepped foot on the streets of Vienna, Austria on 12 October 2019 and made history by being the first athlete to run a marathon in under 2 hours (1 hour 59 minutes and 40 seconds to be precise).

Did he do it barefoot? No. He'd use every technological advantage he could as he wore specialist shoes that naturally encouraged a forefoot running style, efficient running biomechanics and the transfer of kinetic energy in each stride. But had he perfected his technique through barefoot practice as a child on the dirt roads of the Rift Valley which then allowed him to use the technological advantage? Yes.

In summary, I was not Kipchoge or Bikila. In fact, after 157 days at sea I couldn't even be compared to a below-average junior cross-country runner in Africa, since my baby feet were so poorly coordinated and conditioned. This is why each week's training schedule in the Recovery Mesocycle of this book begins with a barefoot, low-intensity steady state run which should be performed (wherever possible) barefoot.[72] Using this ancient form of rehab (that today has become supported by modern sports science) time and distance is irrelevant, since more important is strengthening the intricate muscles of the feet once again, perfecting technique and reviving my long-lost sense of proprioception.

FIT BUT FATIGUED AND STRONG BUT SICK

AUTUMN 2018, LONDON, ENGLAND

It's 9 a.m. on 18 December 2018 in West London. Christmas is a week away which means the country's capital has had its annual festive facelift as every road, path and pedestrianised street becomes illuminated with decorations, mistletoe is hung over every archway and the air is filled with scent of mulled wine and roasted chestnuts. Unfortunately, I couldn't fully enjoy any of this. This is because it's fair to say 2018 hadn't ended well for me, as both my upper body and lower body had been diagnosed as barely functioning. But as the year came to an end, it was about to go from bad to worse as I headed to my final medical meeting on Harley Street. A road famous for its private medical specialists that date back to the nineteenth century, there I would be further prodded and probed to assess the damage the swim had caused to my body. But, needless to say, after the dire diagnosis of my 'squishy sea feet' and shoulder surgery, I wasn't looking forward to the results of my blood and urine samples.

By midday, the medical team were looking at all biological markers to assess my body's response to the chronic stress it had experienced at sea with little to no sleep.[73] This meant:

- Blood tests were taken to monitor testosterone-to-cortisol ratio.[74]
- Urine tests were taken to measure my cortisol-to-cortisone ratio.[75]
- Any variations in heart rate were carefully noted.[76]

Even without the results, I knew I wasn't going to get a glowing report and the frown of empathy upon the doctor's face confirmed it as he gave his diagnosis.

'You're basically very fit, but injured and very fatigued,' he said.

If it was possible to smile and sulk at the same time I probably would have done, since his verdict was a compliment wrapped in bad news.

'Your body is now paying the price for your time at sea.'

'Oh, my shoulder and squishy sea feet?' I asked.

'No, it's not just your musculoskeletal system [relating to muscles, ligaments and tendons and bones]. Your entire body is in a state of chaos since the frequency and intensity of the swim in conjunction with insufficient sleep and recovery has created havoc in the muscle tissue, upset the body's immunity and harassed the delicate balance of the hormonal system [homeostasis].'[77]

What he was describing was overtraining[78] verging on chronic fatigue.[79] This is when your rate of physical exertion is greater than your rate of recovery. While this is the result of many factors and physiological failures within the body, what is essentially happening is the malfunction of the autonomic nervous system as the sympathetic nervous system and parasympathetic nervous system no longer work in harmony.

It sounds complicated, but it's not.

The autonomic system is the part of the peripheral nervous system that controls and regulates the internal organs without conscious effort (i.e. autonomously). Everything from your blood vessels, stomach, intestine, liver, kidneys, bladder, genitals, lungs, pupils, heart, and sweat, salivary and digestive glands are influenced by your autonomic system. It can then be further divided into your:

- **Sympathetic** nervous system.
- **Parasympathetic** nervous system.

Generally, the sympathetic nervous system prepares the body for stressful situations and is responsible for 'fight or flight'. It does this by increasing the heart rate and the force of heart contractions, and widens (dilates) the airways to make breathing easier. It causes the body to release stored energy. Muscular strength is increased. It also causes palms to sweat, pupils to dilate and hairs to stand on end. All while slowing down the processes within the body that are less important in emergencies, such as digestion and urination. Under stress and fuelled by adrenaline, this entire process is considered to be **catabolic** (put simply, the body breaks down).

In contrast, the parasympathetic nervous system handles a lot of our normal 'day-to-day' life since (generally) it's job is to conserve and restore. It slows the heart rate and decreases blood pressure. It stimulates the digestive tract to process food and eliminate wastes. Energy from the processed food is used to restore and build tissues, therefore this entire process is said to be **anabolic** (put simply, the body rebuilds and regrows).

RECOVERY
Parasympathetic Nervous System
Anabolic (builds)
Digests food
Makes hormones
Repairs muscles
State of relaxation

STRESS (EXERCISE)
Catabolic (breaks down)
Increases heart rate
Increase blood pressure
Increases triglycerides
Slows non-essential systems such as digestion and immune function

What happens in healthy (low-stress) individuals is that there's a perfect, synergistic switch between the parasympathetic and sympathetic nervous systems, via a mechanism called the **HPA**

axis. Essentially, during any stressful situation a cocktail of stress hormones is released into the body to bring about well-orchestrated physiological changes that for years have ensured our survival. These physiological changes prime us for either fight or flight (or in this instance sink or swim, freeze or float) and all begin in the brain (see diagram). There follows a carefully orchestrated (near-instantaneous) sequence of hormonal changes that works like this:

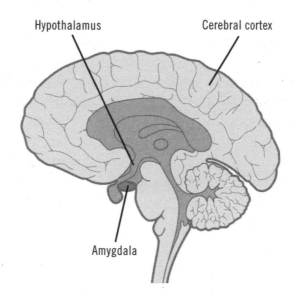

- Our eyes and ears send information to the amygdala (an area of the brain that contributes to emotional processing that we're in trouble).
- The amygdala decides if we're in real danger.
- If we are, it sends a distress signal to the hypothalamus (this area of the brain functions like a command centre which prepares the body through the nervous system for fight or flight).
- It does this by sending a signal to the adrenal glands.
- These glands respond by pumping the hormone epinephrine (also known as adrenaline) into the bloodstream. As epinephrine

circulates through the body, it brings on a number of physiological changes:

- o The heart beats faster and pushes blood to the muscles, heart and vital organs.
- o Pulse, breathing rate and blood pressure go up.
- o Airways in the lungs open to oxygenate the body and brain (increasing alertness).
- o Sight, hearing and other senses become sharper.
- o Blood sugar (glucose) flood into the bloodstream to supply energy to the body.

As the initial surge of epinephrine subsides, the hypothalamus activates the second component of the stress response system, the HPA axis (which also includes the pituitary and adrenal glands). This relies on a series of hormonal signals to keep the sympathetic nervous system – the 'gas pedal' – pressed down and if the brain continues to perceive something as dangerous, adrenal glands are prompted to release cortisol. The body therefore stays 'revved up' and on high alert and only when the threat passes will cortisol levels start to fall.

However, during times of chronic stress (basically the past 157 days I spent at sea) the HPA axis can become de-sensitised to the calming effects of the parasympathetic nervous system, leading to sympathetic nervous system dominance and adrenal overload. This results in the physical, mental and emotional exhaustion experienced in chronic fatigue.

In simpler terms, you're stuck in 'fight or flight' stress mode.

Back in the clinic, the doctor said, 'We see it in military personnel[80] and firefighters[81] too who have been unable to sleep,[82] recover and rest and therefore hormonal and neurologic imbalances result in fatigue, depression, insomnia, irritability and a complete lack of motivation.'

I won't lie, his verdict hit me like a tonne of bricks.

Just days before I was emerging from the sea at Margate as my swim around Great Britain was celebrated, but fast forward 48 hours and I'm being told that I'm fragile, frail and my body is failing.

'Honestly, I'm amazed you're still functioning and not bedridden,' he said.

'Also, are you aware you're missing quite a bit of skin from your tongue and neck?'

'Oh yes, I left most of that around Scotland,' I replied while telling him about the unholy wetsuit chafing and how the salt in the seawater had essentially eroded chunks of my tongue away.

'What about the abrasion scars on your hands and feet?' he asked confused, wondering how I picked up those injuries from the swim.

'Oh, they're not from the swim. They're from when I repeatedly climbed a rope until I scaled the height of Everest for charity.'

Shaking his head in disapproval and disbelief he then asked, 'And dare I ask about the scars on your stomach?'

'Oh, that's from a poorly fitted harness when I pulled a 1.4 tonne car for a marathon. It looks worse than it is, and again we raised so much for charity so I now wear them as badges of honour,' I said still smiling and sulking.

Taking notes while shaking his head, he then asked, 'Is there anything else I need to be aware of?'

I nodded, feeling like a naughty schoolboy. I then started to list my athletic adventures of the last three years:

2016

- January: Ran a marathon (26.2 miles) pulling a 1,400 kg car.
- April: Climbed a 20 m rope (repeatedly) for 19 hours until I'd scaled the height of Everest (8,848 m).
- August: Covered 1,000 miles (barefoot) in a month carrying a 50 kg Marine backpack.

- November: Completed the Nevis Triathlon in the Caribbean carrying a 100 lb tree.

2017

- May: 10 km swim pulling a 100 lb tree in Windermere, England.
- July: 40 km swim pulling a 100 lb tree in Keswick, England.
- November: 100 km swim pulling a 100 lb tree in the Caribbean between St Lucia and Martinique.

2018

- January: 185 km swim (over 48 hours) at the Royal Marines Training Centre in Devon (England).
- June to November: 1,780 mile swim around Great Britain over 157 days.

'Do you know what your next adventure *must* be?' he asked.

'No?' I replied, but keen to hear some ideas.

'Sleep, rest and recover,' he said sternly.

'Oh,' I said, a little disappointed that Everest base camp wasn't on the list.

'I'm being deadly serious, Ross. You're practically elite at everything you do apart from sleeping, resting and recovering. But if you want to continue a life of adventure, you have to take your rehab seriously.'

I stopped to think about what he was saying.

It was true, even now back on land, that I was struggling to adjust back into civilised society and was very aware I had developed some pretty odd habits during my time away. For instance, now no longer spending 12 hours (and 30-plus miles) in the ocean each day, I had to remind myself to:

- Shower regularly.
- Use a proper toilet (not the sea).

- 'Dial back' on the 10,000 calories per day.
- Try to sleep for longer than four hours.

The first three I was managing quite well, but this last one was proving tricky.

You see, during my time at sea I existed in this strange world where my sleep (and therefore recovery) was no longer dictated by the rising and setting of the sun, but instead was governed by the tides that changed every six hours. Basically, I would eat and sleep when the tide was moving against us and swim when it moved in our favour, which meant my brain had been rewired to this form of bi-phasic sleep (sleeping twice a day for a short amount of time).

What's worse is that some days we wouldn't sleep at all.

Crossing the Bristol Channel, Irish Sea and Moray Firth we would swim non-stop for up to 72 hours to make it across before we were hit by storms or ships. What this meant was my sleep was not only deprived but it was also disturbed, and now back on land I would find it impossible to sleep for more than four hours each night. In fact, my brain had been so completely re-wired that on my first night off the boat Hester, my (incredibly patient) girlfriend woke up in the middle of the night to find me sleep-walking around the bedroom in a semi-conscious state looking for my goggles with a strange sense of urgency. Gently guiding me back to bed (with my goggles on my head), she reminded me the swim was over, the tide wasn't changing and there was no need for me to get into the sea.

Silence now filled the room as the doctor opened his laptop and began searching through medical journals related to sleep deprivation. Turning his screen around and drawing my attention to the thousands of pages of research, he drew a parallel between deployment-related insomnia within the military and my sleep issues post swim.

'Hundreds of studies have reported sleep disturbance[83] within the military[84] and have found irregular sleep–wake schedules and adjusting to life back home to be two major contributing factors,' he said. 'Essentially the habits you'd formed at sea (now deeply engrained in your brain) no longer work for you on land as your sleep–wake schedule was completely irregular. Now you need to substitute habits of a relentless work ethic, with habits of routine rest, recovery and rehab.'

Basically, recovery and restorative sleep needed to be my sole focus every day.

How much per night and for how long is hard to determine, since no-one had ever swam 12 hours a day, for 157 days at sea. But scientists from the University of Toronto monitored the sleep patterns of six runners following a 92 km ultra-marathon. Results showed sleep time for each runner 'increased drastically compared to normal sleep patterns on each of the four nights after the marathon', illustrating the body's desperate need for quality sleep to recover.[85]

Using an electroencephalogram (EEG) where electrodes measure brain electrical activity, they specifically found that long periods of 'deep sleep' were induced on the first two nights. This led researchers to conclude this objective and quantitative increase in total sleep time, and particularly 'deep sleep', supports the theory that it is incredibly important for optimal recovery in athletes.

In summary, the *Recovery Mesocycle* is absolutely critical and so often overlooked (I know I've been guilty of this). Which is why I asked the doctor for access to the medical journals on sleep deprivation and got to work. After days, weeks and months of research this is what I learned.

SLEEP–WAKE SCHEDULE

We humans are creatures of habit and we thrive on routine. It's the way we're biologically wired and we've understood this since 350 BCE when Aristotle gave the following (surprising) 'modern' evaluation of sleep and said, 'It is inevitable that every creature which wakes must also be capable of sleeping, since it is impossible that it should continue actualizing its powers perpetually. So, also, it is impossible for any animals to continue always sleeping.'[86]

What he was talking about here was the body's circadian rhythm.[87]

This is your body's inbuilt 'clock' that is responsible for regulating the biological rhythms over a 24-hour period, from the rise and fall of testosterone and cortisol levels to the synchronisation of sleep, wakefulness, mood and cognitive performance.[88]

Worth noting is that the natural cycle of the brain is slightly longer than 24 hours, but it is 'resynchronised' each day by the rising and setting of the sun.[89] This is because the hypothalamus (small part of our brain) that's responsible for body temperature, emotional responses and sexual behaviour among many other things, releases a powerful sleep-inducing hormone called melatonin that drops when we're exposed to sun throughout the day and spikes as it gets darker at night.

Represented in a graph (with an image adapted from world-leading chronobiology experts Michael H Smolensky and Erhard Haus[90]) someone who trains twice a day would likely have a healthy, functioning circadian rhythm like the top chart opposite.

The issue for me was that for 157 days my circadian rhythm was not healthy and functioning.

Instead, it looked like that second chart underneath where my sleep, circadian rhythm and melatonin release was no longer dictated by the rising and setting of the sun, but instead was governed by the tides that changed every six hours.

In the above illustration, you'll notice the (often generous) use of caffeine. Considered to be the most widely consumed psychoactive drug in the world, it's a central nervous system (CNS) stimulant that I used after speaking to friends in the US Navy SEALs who took part in a study that monitored the effects of caffeine on cognitive

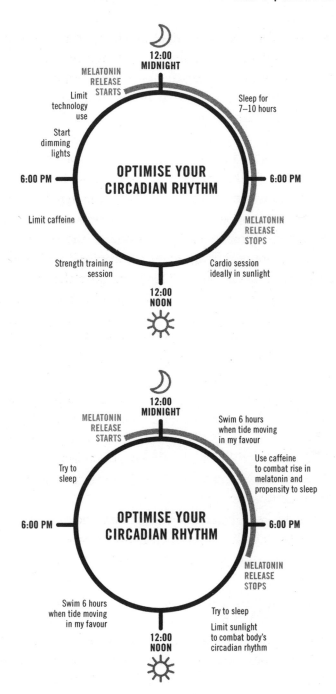

(mental) performance and mood.[91] These Navy Sea–Air–Land trainees volunteered to receive either 100, 200 or 300 mg of caffeine or a placebo in capsule form after 72 hours of sleep deprivation and continuous exposure to other stressors as they performed memory tasks and reaction-time tests.[92]

What the researchers discovered was, 'Caffeine mitigated many adverse effects of exposure to multiple stressors. Caffeine (200 and 300 mg) significantly improved visual vigilance, choice reaction time, repeated acquisition, self-reported fatigue and sleepiness with the greatest effects on tests of vigilance, reaction time, and alertness.' This led them to conclude, 'Even in the most adverse circumstances, moderate doses of caffeine can improve cognitive function, including vigilance, learning, memory, and mood state. When cognitive performance is critical and must be maintained during exposure to severe stress, administration of caffeine may provide a significant advantage. A dose of 200 mg appears to be optimal under such conditions.'

Based on these findings, I decided to supplement the swim with caffeine for the following three reasons:

1. TO COMBAT MY CIRCADIAN RHYTHM

I would use caffeine to try and 'override' the rise in melatonin and the desire to sleep, and essentially 'bio hack' the circadian rhythm. This was based on numerous studies[93] that found that caffeine supplementation[94] can, 'Reverse changes in alertness and mood produced by prolonged sleep deprivation.'[95]

2. TO IMPROVE PERFORMANCE

I would also use caffeine during the swim to outsprint boats when crossing shipping lanes and when rushing to seek safety at a harbour during a storm. Why? Because it's one of the most widely used ergogenic aids (performance-enhancing supplements) permitted by the International Olympic Committee (IOC) since it's been found to 'permit the athlete to train at a greater power output and/or to train longer and has also been shown to increase speed and/or power output in simulated race conditions'.[96]

This was shown across many studies,[97] multiple sports[98] and over various intensities[99] and distances,[100] and all because of the following mechanisms scientists have proposed when researching caffeine and its performance-enhancing properties.[101]

According to many pharmacological reviews in sport (the branch of medicine concerned with the uses, effects and modes of action of drugs)[102] the best-understood mechanisms of caffeine improving performance are based on its ability to:

- **Serve as an 'adenosine blocker'.** Adenosine is one of the more powerful molecules in the body and builds up in the bloodstream during exercise (due to the breakdown of adenosine tri-phosphate (ATP)). This in turn inhibits neural activity, causes drowsiness and essentially tells our body to rest, recover and rebuild our energy reserves. But caffeine was found to attach itself to the same receptors that adenosine would normally latch onto (hence the term 'adenosine blocker') which then reduces adenosine-induced drowsiness. Basically, caffeine serves to lift your foot off the 'biochemical break' of the body that is caused by the increase in adenosine, helping you (in theory) to train harder and longer.

- **Increase your power output.** Research from the *Journal of Medicine and Science in Sport and Exercise* found that caffeine, even when taken in low doses, can improve your power.[103] The study analysed cycling power output and found that a dosage of 3 mg/kg increased power by up to 3.5 per cent when compared to a placebo group. Granted, this might not sound like a lot, but it could be responsible for the new one rep max you put up on the bench press.

- **Improve the 'ionic environment' within the muscle.** Research conducted at the University of Guelph in Ontario, Canada found that caffeine supplementation could 'permit an athlete to train at a greater power output and/or to train longer by producing a more favourable ionic environment within the active muscle.'[104] It's believed it does this by increasing levels of intracellular calcium in skeletal muscle, which in turn makes the muscles contract more efficiently by improving something called 'excitation–contraction coupling'. This is the sequence of events through which the nerve fibre stimulates the skeletal muscle fibre causing its contraction.

3. TO REDUCE PERCEPTION TO PAIN

Numerous studies[105] have shown that caffeine is capable of decreasing pain[106] and perceived level of exertion[107] especially in endurance athletes. As well as serving as an 'adenosine blocker', it enables excitatory neurotransmitters (chemical signals in the brain) such as dopamine, acetylcholine and serotonin to move about more freely and stimulate the brain and therefore 'overrides' feelings of discomfort.[108] Researchers from the Department of Clinical Neurosciences at the University of Oxford concluded, 'The addition of caffeine ($\geq$ 100 mg) provides a small but important increase in the proportion of participants who experience a good level of pain relief.'[109]

There are of course downsides to five months of severe sleep deprivation and such large and 'generous' dosages of caffeine, and I wouldn't recommend it to anyone. This is because you're basically causing an orchestra of biochemical reactions in the body in pursuit of a short-term goal, but that is not sustainable. It's like borrowing money from the bank: it's great at the time, but at some point you will have to pay it back since no-one can survive 'biochemical bankruptcy' for long. So for now, back on land, I had to continue researching rest and studying sleep to create an efficient *Recovery Mesocycle*.

STUDY OF SLEEP

Sleep is, and always will be, absolutely crucial to our survival. The renowned sleep pioneer Allan Rechtschaffen noted that, 'If sleep does not serve an absolutely vital function, then it is the biggest mistake the evolutionary process ever made.'[110] In other words, it would have made no sense for our Palaeolithic ancestors to spend six to eight hours per day sleeping and unconscious, making them vulnerable to predators, unable to hunt, eat and survive . . . unless it was an essential biological function.

What is that function?

Modern researchers don't know exactly and have said, 'Sleep has been one of the mysteries of biology' with many theories proposed.[111] But what we do know, based on hundreds of studies on the patho-physiological consequences of sleep deprivation, is without it we become ill, psychotic and could even die.

This is no exaggeration. In 1894, Russian scientist Marie de Manaceine started experimenting on puppies to test the effects of sleep deprivation. After 4 to 5 days (96 to 120 hours) she reported irreparable lesions in the brain before they all died.[112] The same unfortunate result was found in 1989 with older, larger dogs too, as Italian scientists Lamberto Daddi and Giulio Tarozzi kept them awake for 9 to 17 days before they died.[113]

Obviously (and thankfully) for ethical reasons professional researchers have never pushed the sleep deprivation process beyond this point with human subjects. However, there are horror stories from years ago where sleep deprivation was used as a form of torture. Tracing its origins back to the fifteenth century, an Italian lawyer and doctor by the name of Hippolytus de Marsiliis was the first person to document sleep deprivation as a means of torture.

Discovering it particularly effective because it attacks the deep biological functions at the core of a person's mental and physical health, it was later adopted and adapted by 'witch hunters' in Europe and North America who called this *tortura insomniae* and used it to interrogate thousands of innocent women for alleged sorcery. American historian Andrew Dickson wrote, 'In this way, temporary delusion became chronic insanity, mild cases became violent, torture and death ensued.'[114]

Basically, your own brain will begin to betray you.

Of course, the same happens in extreme sports too, if not to that level. Take the Ultra-Trail du Mont-Blanc (UTMB), for example.[115] Considered one of the most difficult foot races in the world, it's approximately 171 km (106 miles) in distance with a total elevation gain of around 10,040 m (32,940 ft) and crosses the Alps through France, Italy and Switzerland. While the best runners complete the loop in slightly more than 20 hours, most runners take 32 to 46 hours to reach the finish and will have to run throughout two nights in order to complete the race. As a result, hallucinations (perceptual distortions[116]) are common and can take many forms.

All things considered, scientists believe, 'Sleep is an important component of homeostasis, vital for our survival and sleep disorders are associated with significant behavioural and health consequences.'[117] So as we blissfully drift into a slumber our:

- Muscles, tendons and ligaments repair and regrow.
- Neurotransmitters – the chemical signals in the brain – are replenished to keep us motivated, focused and functioning.
- Rejuvenating hormones like human growth hormone (HGH) begin to naturally peak.

This last point is particularly important since HGH is a peptide hormone that stimulates cell reproduction, cell regeneration, growth and recovery. Which is why for all the energy bars and recovery shakes in the world, if you suspect you're overtraining and under-recovered, one of the best things you can do is head to bed.

We've known this as far back as 1968 when research published in the *Journal of Clinical Investigation* stated, 'Sleep results in a major peak of growth hormone secretion.'[118]

It's basic biological 'house maintenance' and athletes can't function without it.[119]

Further to this, research conducted at Stanford University analysed the impact sleeping 10 hours a night had on basketball players' performance after 5 to 7 weeks. Previously, the players had only been sleeping 6 to 9 hours and what the sleep scientists found was their performance dramatically improved.[120]

Not just a little, either. 'Shooting accuracy improved, with free throw percentage increasing by 9 per cent and 3-point field goal percentage increasing by 9.2 per cent,' and, 'Subjects also reported improved overall ratings of physical and mental wellbeing during practices and games.' It concluded that, 'Improvements in specific measures of basketball performance after sleep extension indicate that optimal sleep is likely beneficial in reaching peak athletic performance.'

So where does this nocturnal magic come from? According to research published in *Frontiers in Systems Neuroscience*, it's closely related to our previously mentioned neurotransmitters.[121] Neurotransmitters are the chemicals that work to transmit signals from a neuron to a target cell across a synapse within the body. Pretty much every function within the body is controlled or impacted on by neurotransmitters, from emotional states to mental performance and our perception to fatigue and pain. They are the brain's little chemical messengers and if they are not working correctly due to lack of sleep you can't expect to run, swim, cycle or compete to the best of your ability.

In summary, never underestimate your need for sleep. If you do (based on hundreds of studies in sleep deprivation) you will be physically tired,[122] mentally exhausted,[123] not optimally recovering[124] and the decisions you make will be flawed and impaired.[125]

So how do you get better at sleep during your *Recovery Macrocycle*? Put simply, you must schedule it according to the natural laws that govern human biology. This is something that I learned to do in the African outback where I spent time with the San Bushmen, the last of the great hunter-gatherer civilisations.

A BEDTIME STORY BENEATH THE STARS

It was 20 August 2008 in Namibia, Africa. Woefully underprepared, badly unequipped and with a terrible grasp of the locally spoken dialect, I was learning to hunt on the sun-bleached African plains with the Ju-Wasi tribe. Considered one of the greatest hunter-gatherer civilisations to have ever existed, their way of life closely resembled that of our ancient ancestors and had remained unchanged for thousands of years. As a result, it's fair to assume (based on evolutionary medicine) that the Ju-Wasi were living by the laws that Mother Nature laid out for us humans.

How? Well, their lives were simple with no complications. They hunted and harvested during the day and slept and rested during the night, and everything in between was scheduled according to the rising and setting of the sun.

As an odd, visiting Englishman who'd been welcomed into the village, I have to be honest, I loved their way of life. In fact, having graduated from university a year before, I found both my body and brain appreciated the newly imposed sense of simplicity, as I no longer had to stay up all night revising by artificial light or abruptly interrupt my sleep with an alarm clock to attend morning lectures.

Instead, free from many trappings of modern society, I had been sleeping like a baby in the mud hut that my hosts had built for me. But today was different; we had embarked on a 100-mile hunt across the Namibian wilderness and as the sun began to set in the sky we found ourselves miles from the comfort and safety of the village.

Turning to my newly adopted Ju-Wasi family, I asked what the plan of action was and gesturing with my hands where we'd be sleeping tonight. Communicating among themselves in an ancient language that consisted of clicking sounds and maps drawn in the sand with a stick, I had absolutely no idea what was being said. Fortunately, help was at hand and it came in the form of Tau, my San Bushman brother, who spoke a little English and had adopted me and taken me under his wing.

'What's going on?' I whispered to Tau, not wanting to interrupt.

'They're deciding what to do with you,' he replied.

'Eh? What do you mean, "Do with me?"' I exclaimed.

Tau laughed. He loved winding me up.

'Basically, Duee thinks it will be good for you to sleep out here on your own. It's how you say in your country, "a rites of passage" and all young San Bushmen must learn to do this.'

I turned to Duee who nodded affirmatively.

He was the head of the Ju-Wasi tribe. Standing 5 ft 6 in he was slim, svelte and had deeply indented wrinkle lines engrained into his face from years of hunting in the scorching dry seasons. Each crease and crinkle in the skin almost served as a physical representation of his years of experience as the most esteemed hunter in all of Namibia. Basically, he was so wise and respected that whatever he said was never questioned. Therefore, if he said I had to sleep under the stars on my own, that's exactly what I was going to do.

Moments later and as the sun began to set, I was being shown to my bed for the night that was in the form of a small bush sitting at the base of a cactus tree. Yes, it wasn't exactly comfortable, but to be honest after covering 40 miles today on the hunt I didn't mind and could have fallen asleep anywhere.

Duee then instructed Tau to tell me that I should remain alert throughout the night for predators or anything territorial that might not like a strange Englishman sleeping in their back garden. I nodded and told them I'd see them in the morning, when I'd earned my stripes and could emerge a fully-fledged San Bushman.

Or at least that was my intention.

At first, it was going well. As instructed, my senses were on high alert. I could hear every blade of grass blowing in the wind and see every tree, plant and shrub for miles as they remained partially illuminated by the fading light. But as the sun completely disappeared over the horizon, this is when the problems started to occur.

Not unpleasant problems. In fact, far from it, these were problems of a blissful nature. For me, the peace and quiet I found in the Namibian desert that night was unlike anything I'd ever experienced before. So incredibly quiet that you could almost hear your own heartbeat, and the air was so pure and void of pollution. In fact, everything overhead appeared so clear and close that you could see a shooting star almost every few minutes.

Unfortunately, all of this didn't help when I was trying to remain alert for angry lions, packs of hyenas or frisky rhinos during mating season. Instead, I found myself happily using the base of the cactus as a pillow, as I lay on my back and gazed up at the sky before (accidentally) drifting off into one of the best nights of sleep that I've ever had.

Hours passed and as night turned to day and the sun rose in the sky, I was woken by Duee, Tau and my Bushmen brothers standing over me.

'Were you asleep?' Tau asked, shaking his head disapprovingly.

With my eyes still closed, I realised I had messed up royally and that Duee and my Bushmen brothers wouldn't be happy at my failed attempt to stay awake and alert.

'No, I'm not asleep. I'm resting my eyes while my other senses are on duty.'

Unconvinced, Tau translated for the others who all burst out laughing.

'You might want to check your other senses,' he said. 'Because they clearly failed to pick up on the animal that was circling you as you slept.'

Duee then pointed to a set of footprints just metres away from where I'd been sleeping. He wasn't lying either; it seemed that through the night something had come to investigate what the strange creature, new to Namibia, was doing snoring into a cactus.

I apologised and breathed a giant sigh of relief.

It seems my Bushmen skills were awful, but my ability to sleep on a cactus was incredible. But why was I able to drift into such a deep sleep despite sleeping on a pillow of pins while being inspected by the African wildlife?

Well, that's (again) related to your circadian rhythm which should make scheduling sleep easy. That's because it's a natural law that governs our biology, yet research estimates that over one-third of the adult population in the USA sleeps less than the recommended minimum of seven hours per night.[126] This 'seven-hour rule' wasn't just plucked out of the air, but was decided upon after a panel of experts[127] reviewed over 5,000 scientific studies[128] relating to sleep deprivation[129] and found it was strongly correlated with shorter lifespans[130] and a whole list of health conditions like obesity,[131] diabetes[132] and cardiovascular disease,[133] to name but a few.[134]

So, what's happening?

You see, ever since Thomas Edison invented the lightbulb (his final patent being filed on 4 November 1879) we have been increasingly capable of manipulating our environments with artificial light which in turn interferes with our sleep–wake cycle (circadian rhythm) as we become less dependent on the sun for light. As a result, our brain (hypothalamus) and the release of melatonin no longer runs like clockwork as nature intended and the result is what many experts believe to be a, 'Public health epidemic that is often unrecognized, under-reported.'[135]

But the lightbulb isn't solely to blame; our lack of sleep is also a cultural issue too. We're taught from an early age that the 'early bird catches the worm' and the more hours you're awake the more motivated you appear to be. Productivity and sleep deprivation are therefore related, and obesity and poor mental health are closely related 'cousins'.

But out in Namibia, I was free from this.

My body, brain and biology was able to work the way in which my circadian rhythm was designed. So, in 2019, I took the lessons of Namibia and tried to replicate them in order to optimise rest and recovery. Essentially, re-scheduling my day, resynchronising my circadian rhythm and re-writing my habits by following these *6 Steps to Better Sleep:*

1. MORNING SUN SETS YOUR 'BODY CLOCK'

Studies show morning sunlight reinforces your natural circadian rhythm, by signalling to your brain that bedtime is over, it's time to suppress melatonin, increase cortisol production and attack the day. Researchers claim, 'These hormones can be considered to be stable markers of the circadian time structure and therefore useful tools to validate rhythms' synchronisation of human subjects.'[136]

2. LEARN TO 'DIGITAL DETOX'

In the modern digital age, experts stress the need to manage the amount of light you're pumping into your eyes from electronic devices in the evening. This is because studies show, 'Modern light exposure patterns contribute to late sleep schedules and disrupt sleep and circadian clocks'[137] by delaying the release of melatonin.

3. REDUCE CAFFEINE INTAKE

Research reveals there is a strong association between daily intake of caffeine[138] and reduced sleep quality and quantity[139] since consumption causes a reduction in 6-sulfatoxymelatonin (main metabolite of melatonin) which interferes with our natural sleep–wake cycle.[140] Obviously effects vary from person to person,[141] but studies show even if taken six hours before bed, a small cup of coffee can have disruptive effects on sleep.[142]

4. TRAIN TO SLEEP

In 2007, a study published in the *Journal of Neuroscience* wrote, 'The present suggest that depletion of cerebral energy stores and accumulation of the sleep promoting substance adenosine after exercise[143] may play a key role in homeostatic sleep regulation.'[144] Put simply, train like an animal during the day and sleep like a baby at night. Also, studies reveal that the type of exercise doesn't even matter;[145] everything from strength training to yoga was shown to have sleep-enhancing benefits.[146]

5. FIND 65°F (18.3°C)

Researchers found, 'The thermal environment (temperature of the room) is one of the most important factors that can affect sleep.'[147] This has been supported by numerous studies over the years, but a large-scale analysis of 765,000 survey respondents found that most people experience abnormal sleeping patterns during the hotter summer months.[148] This is why scientists claim the perfect room temperature is between 60°F and 67°F (15.6°C and 19.4°C). This is because your body's internal temperature changes during a 24-hour period with your circadian rhythm, but if the room temperature is too hot or cold it may cause circadian rhythm malfunctions and therefore disrupt sleep.

6. SUPPLEMENT YOUR SLEEP

This final tip could be the proverbial cherry on top of your night-time (figuratively and literally). This is because cherries are one food known to be naturally high in melatonin, which research published in the *European Journal of Nutrition*[149] found increases melatonin levels and serotonin levels which in turn improved the quality and quantity of their sleep.

AUTUMN | RECOVERY TRAINING PLAN

Science-based and stripped back to allow optimal time to recover, firstly, remember this is strength training rehab. The goal is not to lift Herculean weights or run a marathon PB; the goal is to re-acquire lost skill, strength and function with an emphasis on rest and recovery. It does this by fusing different training methods into a hybrid training programme that takes inspiration from:

- Ancient and modern sports rehabilitation practices.
- Low-intensity steady state training.
- Bodyweight and resistance band conditioning.
- Simple multi-limb powerlifting movements.

Together, these helped to redevelop lost and forgotten movement patterns and rebuilt my body from the ground up.

RECOVERY & REHAB STRENGTH: THE FORMAT

The strength workouts themselves are biomechanically divided. This means 'push', 'pull' and 'lower body' movements are performed in different sessions which encourages lots of big, functional movements that use universal motor recruitment patterns to develop neurological efficiency. It's also inspired by the simplicity of a powerlifting programme. This is because the squat, bench and deadlift are considered the 'backbone' of many strength and conditioning routines and powerlifting is a time-efficient, safe, multi-limb strength training protocol to apply weight, stress and stimuli to the body's structures (bones, muscles, joints, ligaments or tendons) for them to adapt, improve and become more resilient.

Equally important to remember is the intensity, volume and frequency of training is kept low, allowing enough time to recover, repair and rehab, and most importantly never (under any circumstances) struggle and 'grind out' a repetition or train to failure. This is a *Recovery Mesocycle* where the body is in a delicate state, therefore we don't want to tax the body too much and overtrain. But more importantly, science shows we don't have to if our goal is to rebuild strength within the muscles, joints and ligaments. Research published in the *British Journal of Sports Medicine* stated that, 'Fatigue does not appear to be critical stimuli for strength gain, and resistance training can be effective without the severe discomfort and acute physical effort associated with fatiguing contractions.'[150] This was supported by the *Scandinavian Journal of Medicine Science in Sports* which found, 'Repetition failure is not critical to elicit significant neural and structural changes to skeletal muscle.'[151]

REPETITIONS & WEIGHT

Drilling down into the specifics, the strength programme in this book mainly works within 8 to 12 repetitions with 80 per cent to 70 per cent of your one-repetition maximum (1RM). For those not familiar with this, central to any strength programme is knowing your one-repetition maximum (i.e. the maximum amount of weight you can lift just once). When you know this number for a particular lift, you're able to calculate the amount of repetitions you can perform with a certain weight based on the table below. To keep things simple, if you bench press 100 kg for 1-repetition then you should be able to perform 4-repetitions with 90 kg, 8-repetitions with 80 kg and so on. Some workouts are set up differently. They might detail the number of repetitions you should be performing. That's fine, instead you look at the number of repetitions and then use the corresponding percentage of your 1RM. You're simply using the table below to do the conversion in a slightly different way.

Calculate Your One-Rep Max (1RM)	
Repetitions	% One-Rep Max (1RM)
1	100
2	95
3	93
4	90
5	87
6	85
7	83
8	80
9	77
10	75
11	73
12	70

*Remember that each exercise has its own 1RM.
**These are only estimates. The lower your rep count, the more accurate your 1RM estimate will be.

It's important to note the reason the programme doesn't strictly state the exact repetitions (and weight) and instead 'loosely' recommends 8 to 12 repetitions is because the entire programme requires you to train intuitively. What this means is that if you know attempting 12 repetitions will require you to strain and struggle, then don't and drop the weight at 10 or 11 repetitions. Essentially, empower yourself and become your own best expert, since no-one knows your body better than you.

RECOVERY TRAINING PLAN (AUTUMN): MICROCYCLE (WEEK'S PLAN)

This microcycle includes FIVE sessions per week which consists of:

- THREE strength-based rehab routines that use ancient and modern rehab to re-build the durability of the muscles, ligaments and tendons.
- TWO endurance-based rehab routines that are low intensity and no more than 45 minutes long to aid recovery, enhance sleep strategies and improve the resilience of the body in its entirety.

Worth restating is the focus of the entire mesocycle is *Recovery . . .* never fatigue.

The volume and intensity of training is kept low and all efforts are focused on restoring the stability, strength and function of the joints, ligaments, smaller intricate muscles and the health of the body in its entirety. Represented in a table a week's training looks like this:

	Monday	Tuesday	Wednesday
SESSION	Barefoot Run	'Pull' Routine	Leg Routine
PURPOSE	*Endurance-Based Prehab/Rehab*	*Strength-Based Prehab/Rehab*	*Strength-Based Prehab/Rehab*

Thursday	Friday	Saturday	Sunday
'Push' Routine	Barefoot Run	REST	REST
Strength-Based Prehab/Rehab	*Endurance-Based Prehab/Rehab*	*REST*	*REST*

5-DAY REHAB STRENGTH: THE PROGRAMME

MONDAY & FRIDAY:

LOW-INTENSITY STEADY STATE BAREFOOT RUN

Exercises	Time	Distance	Speed
Barefoot Run	20–60 minutes	Irrelevant	Irrelevant

Coaching Cues

There is no single 'perfect running form' since everyone's body is different, but understand there are some common traits in movement patterns among elite runners. Based on these, here's some coaching cues to help: first, focus on a relaxed, soft landing as you forefoot strike during each stride. After the front of your foot lands, let the heel down gradually, bringing the foot and lower leg to a gentle landing as you dorsiflex your ankle under the control of your calf muscles. It's like when you land from a jump, flexing the hip, knee and ankle. Again, the landing should feel soft, springy and comfortable. Do not overstride (land with your foot too far in front of your hips). Overstriding while forefoot or midfoot striking requires you to point your toe more than necessary, adding stress to the calf muscles, Achilles tendon and the arch of the foot. It often feels as if your feet are striking the ground beneath your hips. When barefoot running (with increased proprioception) you will be better able to tell where and how hard you're landing on your feet.

TUESDAY: 'PULL' TRAINING

Exercises	Repetitions	Sets	Rest
Passive Hang (Brachiating) (p 301)	30–45 seconds	3	90 seconds
Dynamic Hanging (p 302)	10 (each side)	3	90 seconds
Scapula Pull-Ups (p 302)	10	3	90 seconds
Pull-Ups (pronated) (p 303) (Optional: Weighted)	10	3	90 seconds
Spider Bicep Curls (p 305)	12	3	60 seconds
Farmer's Walk (p 306)	10 metres forward then 10 metres back	3	45 seconds

WEDNESDAY: LEG ROUTINE

Exercises	Repetitions	Sets	Rest
Seated (box) Squats (p 312)	8–12	3	90 seconds
Front Seated Squats (p 311)	8–10	3	90 seconds
(Dumbbell) Weighted Lunges (p 312)	10 metres (forward) 4 (each leg)	3	60 seconds
Barbell Standing Barefoot Calf (Toe) Raises (p 313)	8–12	3	90 seconds

THURSDAY: 'PUSH' TRAINING

Exercises	Repetitions	Sets	Rest
External rotation with band (p 320)	8–12	3	90 seconds
Internal rotation with band (p 320)	8–12	3	90 seconds
Scapula Push-Ups (p 319)	8–12	3	90 seconds
Barbell Bench Press (p 322)	8–12	3	90 seconds
Dumbbell Shoulder Press (p 322)	8–12	3	90 seconds
Tricep Pushdowns (p 323)	8–12	3	60 seconds

WINTER | BASE
MESOCYCLE OVERVIEW

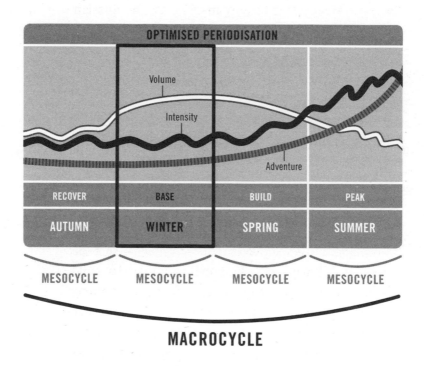

OPTIMISED PERIODISATION

Volume

Intensity

Adventure

| RECOVER | BASE | BUILD | PEAK |
| AUTUMN | WINTER | SPRING | SUMMER |

MESOCYCLE | MESOCYCLE | MESOCYCLE | MESOCYCLE

MACROCYCLE

'SOMETIMES YOU HAVE TO TRAIN TO TRAIN'

Firstly, notice the volume of training is high, but the intensity is low.

The goal is *not* to set new personal bests (that will come later) but rather to improve work capacity (habituate stress) which is the body's ability to perform and positively tolerate training of a given intensity or duration and build a solid athletic (aerobic) base.

The reason this is so important is because *'sometimes you have to train to train'*. What this mean is you have to build a certain 'athletic base' and work capacity to tolerate harder, heavier or more intense sessions later. You simply can't go from 5 hours training per week (during the *Recovery Mesocycle*) to 20+ hours per week (like most elite Ironman triathletes) since it will be too much stress for the body to handle.

The *Base Mesocycle* is heavily inspired by the Russian Conjugate Sequence System (CJSS) and General Physical Preparedness (GPP). This was a system of training developed in the Soviet Union in the late 1960s and early 1970s. If viewed from a macrocycle perspective, the CJSS was conducted over many years (not just one) where young athletes were entered into specialist sport schools[152] to try and identify the next Michael Phelps, Usain Bolt or Serena Williams. Although traditionally associated with the old Eastern Bloc[153] countries,[154] today similar systems can be found in China[155] where the goal is to:

- **Develop General Physical Preparedness (GPP).** Children are encouraged to develop a variety of skills that are not specific to a sport (run, jump, swim, climb and throw) but that build an athlete's work capacity, motor skills (movement), strength, speed, stamina and skill all at once, which they can later use to:
- **Develop Specific Physical Preparedness (SPP).** As the youngsters develop they may demonstrate certain physical attributes of strength, speed or stamina that could mean they are biologically destined to excel in a certain sport. So (through systematic identification[156]) the best young athletes are given access to coaches, gyms and resources to foster this talent[157] so they can become elite-level sprinters, swimmers or gymnasts (this is what we develop later in the *Build Mesocycle*).

This became known in Russia as the Process of Achieving Sports Mastery (PASM).[158] Rooted in the research of A Novikov and N G Ozolin (considered the 'fathers of Russian physical education'),[159] what's interesting is during the initial GPP stage the amount of sport-specific exercise is limited and constitutes only 5–10 per cent of the total training volume, in order to avoid specialising too early.[160] This is based on the results of an experimental longitudinal study from the former East Germany[161] and a descriptive longitudinal survey regarding youth developmental programmes from the former USSR[162] that found over a 14-year period a multilateral training regimen is superior in the early stages of development and promotes a strong, stable foundation for athletic success (see table).

Early specialisation	Multilateral programme
Performance improvements were immediate	Performance improvements were continuous
Best performances between 15–16 because of early adaptation	Best performances over 18 due to physical and mental maturation
Performances inconsistencies within competition	Performance consistencies within competitions
By 18, many athletes quite or 'burnout'	After 18, many athletes were starting to 'come into their own'
Forced adaptation accounted for a high rate of injuries	Gradual adaptation accounted for a low rate of injuries

'This provides the base framework for the neurological construction of all subsequently developed motor skills.'
The Development of the Russian Conjugate Sequence System[163]

The theory underlying this system was that if an athlete developed a well-rounded athletic base, their overall motor potential and their ability to move would correspondingly improve. Over time, you can then specialise with this newly developed neurological efficiency and play any sport. Without it, you will be forever training with the 'physiological handbrake' on.

They believed the direct relationship between the central nervous system (CNS) and physical training played a paramount role in an athlete's adaptation to training. The idea being that if they were neurologically efficient at a young age, they would be able to mature and develop through the different stages of the PASM framework.

This is why the National Strength and Conditioning Association states, 'The major emphasis is establishing a base level of conditioning to increase the athlete's tolerance for more intense training. Conditioning activities begin at relatively low intensities and high volumes; long-slow distance running or swimming: low intensity plyometric and high repetition resistance training with light to moderate resistances.'[164] It adds, 'Because high-volume training causes significant fatigue and can involve large time commitments, the athlete is not exposed to optimal conditions for improving sport-specific technique. As a result, technique training is not a high priority during this period [and can come at a later date within the macrocycle].'

So why is this all relevant to me?

Since I am not a 9-year-old sporting hopeful from Russia in the 1960s and 1970s, but a 34-year-old Englishman whose muscles has been shrivelled and shrunk at sea. In view of my fragile physiology, I basically had to go 'back to school'. Also, research shows GPP can play an important role, 'as active rest, assisting the restoration processes after significant, specific loading and counteracting the monotony of the training.'[165]

Through the winter, I would begin my *Base Mesocycle* and my goals would become focused on:

- **Developing Ancient Spartan Strength.** Replicating the conditions that made the Spartan Army so feared and revered by implementing a form of adversity training that sharpens the mind and hardens the body.

- **Endurance-Based General Physical Preparedness**. To build work capacity, I ran laps of a 5 km obstacle course to build an aerobic base ('gas tank').
- **Strength-Based General Physical Preparedness**. Also to build work capacity, in the form of a mile run pushing a (small) tractor coupled with tyre flips, keg carries and sledge hammers hits on the farmyard.
- **Habituating Stress.** Through ice swimming and adventure-based askēsis, so psychologically and physiologically I am able to positively tolerate training that's higher in intensity and longer in volume (work capacity).

This final point is so important, but so often overlooked. This is why it's become a tradition of mine to start every year's *Base Mesocycle* with an ice swim to 'wash away' any spiritual decay as I start to habituate the stress caused by a higher volume and intensity of training. It's one of the best forms of adventure-based askēsis and healthy hardship, and is inspired by the ancient Greek army's concept of 'getting wintered'.

BASE MESOCYCLE: START WITH A SWIM

WINTER 2019, MANLEY MERE, ENGLAND

It's 7 a.m. on 18 January 2019 in Cheshire, England. After weeks of routine rest and rehab (of the barefoot and brachiating variety) my *Recovery Mesocycle* had come to an end and I no longer owned a pair of squishy sea feet or battered rotator cuffs. Now I was eager to begin my next phase of training and build a solid athletic foundation with a well-programmed *Base Mesocycle*, which would begin at

Manley Mere, a lakeside water sports centre and adventure park that's owned by good friends of mine (Alistair and Kate). It had been converted from their family's dairy farm in 1984 and was nestled among 40 acres of fields in the English countryside. Equipped with a huge lake to swim in, an adventure trail to run across and an old farmyard full of equipment to perform old-style strongman training with, today there was a thin layer of frost covering the ground which meant the water temperature dipped below 2°C (35.6°F). These were the perfect conditions to habituate stress and get 'wintered'.

This is an idea that should be central to everyone's *Base Mesocycle* and is inspired by the ancient Greek philosopher Epictetus who advocated a period of cold, hard and brutal training for soldiers as they prepared for war. He famously said, 'We must undergo a hard winter training and not rush into things for which we haven't prepared' because so often wars were not fought in the winter in ancient Greece, therefore this time should be spent training and preparing for battles that could come in spring. Of course, normally I use this idea of becoming 'battle ready' in the figurative sense, but for today's session I did mean it quite literally. For I would be joined by my good friend Eddie Hall, the 2017 world's strongest man who was preparing to make his boxing debut the following year. He too was at the start of his *Base Mesocycle*, so we agreed to meet up and train in the sub-zero temperatures wearing nothing but trunks and a smile as we habituated stress together.

Entering into the water that day, I must admit I was nervous. Although Eddie was a very accomplished swimmer in his youth, winter swimming is a completely different sport and if anything went wrong I'm not sure conventional lifesaving techniques apply to a man weighing 28 stone (177.8 kg) and standing 6 ft 3 in (1.92 m) tall. This is why I was so keen to communicate all the dangers we would face today as we waded into the lake up to our waists. But before I could get into the science of ice swimming, it became immediately obvious that the sensation was foreign to Eddie's physiology and was something his genitals didn't like.

'Oh no . . . I can't feel my testicles,' he said with genuine unease.

'But I don't understand why you need to feel them right now?' I replied laughing.

'No, no, I'm being serious. Can you get frostbite on your penis?' he asked.

'Hmm . . . I'd be surprised,' I said.

'Surprised? But you're not saying "no" entirely,' he continued to quiz me with concern.

In many ways, it was a fair question. Also as a sea swimmer and sports scientist who's swum in some of the world's coldest environments, I'd coincidentally come across research on this very topic. So I told him that although it's a rare occurrence, studies show it is possible (in theory) since seawater freezes at −1.9°C and human tissue at −0.55°C.[166]

I then assured him that because we were in a freshwater lake that's just above freezing, that whatever he was feeling in his trunks wasn't frostbite and that the safety and wellbeing of his penis was actually low down on the list of dangers surrounding ice swimming.

'If the safety of my shlong is a low priority, do I want to know what you consider high?' he asked.

Inviting him to walk deeper into the lake, I then listed the three biggest dangers that everyone must understand when ice swimming:

DANGER 1: 'COLD SHOCK' | Time: 0–10 seconds. The biggest factor that accounts for most cold-water deaths is 'cold shock'. According to research published in the *British Journal of Sports Medicine*,[167] 'This is a physiological response of a gasp and uncontrollable hyperventilation, initiated by the dynamic response of the cutaneous cold receptors, resulting in the aspiration of the small volume of water necessary to initiate the drowning process.'[168] Basically, you panic, hyperventilate and start drowning.

DANGER 2: HYPOTHERMIA | Time: 20–30 minutes. Hypothermia occurs when your body loses heat faster than it can produce heat, causing a dangerously low body temperature. Obviously, there are many factors that will impact on how susceptible a person is to hypothermia, but progressive signs and symptoms are as follows:

- 37°C (core) temperature: Your body functions as normal.
- 36°C (core) temperature: Shivering.
- 35°C (core) temperature: Confusion, disorientation and introversion.
- 34°C (core) temperature: Amnesia.
- 33°C (core) temperature: Cardiac arrhythmias.
- 33°C–30°C (core) temperature: Clouding of consciousness.
- 30°C (core) temperature: Loss of consciousness.
- 28°C (core) temperature: Ventricular fibrillation.
- 25°C (core) temperature: Death.

Interestingly, these figures are often cited as science-backed estimates. Since although the core body temperature associated with death is often quoted as 25°C, the lowest temperature recorded (to date) after accidental exposure to cold water (with a full recovery) was a body temperature of 13.7°C (56.6°F).[169]

DANGER 3: 'AFTER DROP' | Time: 60 minutes+. The mistake many people make is thinking they're safe once they've exited the water, but the truth is they must be very cautious of another physiological phenomenon called 'after drop'.[170] When you are submerged in cold water, your body reduces blood flow to the skin and extremities (arms, legs, hands and feet) through something called 'peripheral vasoconstriction' and increases blood flow to the core to protect your vital organs. This is an innate self-preservation mechanism that occurs to ensure we retain heat and can survive in cold water longer.[171] But as you exit the water and start to warm up, this process is reversed and the blood starts to leave your core and vital organs and recirculate back to your extremities and peripheral blood vessels, cooling as it travels. As a result, you can lose up to 4.5°C from your core temperature[172] which in turn can cause you to shiver, develop hypothermia or lose consciousness.[173] What's worse is that studies show if you attempt to rush this process of re-warming by having a warm shower, you risk warm blood (that has pooled in your core) returning to your hands and feet at speed, leading to rapid cooling. This is why it was so important the team warmed up slowly and gradually.

Finally, studies show that if you're able to do all of the above in a safe manner and systematically subject your body to lower temperatures and longer immersion in the cold, then you train your body (and brain's) ability to habituate stress.

HABITUATE STRESS

Habituation is a psychological learning process where there is a decrease in response to a stimulus after being repeatedly exposed to it. It sounds complicated, but it's not. It means any stressor you're exposed to (whether it be psychological or physiological) provokes a stress response. However, the more times you're exposed to it the less stressful it becomes.

It was first described in the landmark paper by R F Thompson and W A Spencer in 1966 entitled 'Habituation: A model phenomenon for the study of neuronal substrates of behaviour'[174] but has since been expanded upon to find habituation causes a variety of responses in the body and mind which can influence behaviour.

One of these responses is related to our fight-or-flight response and the release of hormones, since it has been known that, 'The magnitude of hypothalamic–pituitary–adrenal (HPA) activation occurring in response to a stressor declines with repeated exposure to that same stressor.'[175]

This explains why scientists found karate fighters with three years of experience had a greater control over their stress hormone release compared to untrained subjects. Researchers found, 'Long-term karate practice is associated with a significant modulation of stress hormones.'[176]

Now, these are only preliminary results and while some studies show most people's stress response decreases the more times they're exposed to something psychologically stressful, for some it does not change or even increases. This is largely based on your *subjective* evaluation of the situation, sport or adventure and the level of stress.[177]

'The latest studies indicate that the neuroendocrine response to competition depends more on subjective factors related to the cognitive evaluation of the situation.'
Neuroscience & Bio-Behavioural Reviews (2005)

Let's take skydiving, for example. Research published in *Frontiers of Human Neuroscience* stated that, 'It is uncertain whether stress reactivity habituates to this stressor given that skydiving remains a risky, life-threatening challenge with every jump despite experience.'[178] But, 'Results suggest that experience may modulate the coordination of emotional response with cortisol reactivity to skydiving' and, 'Alters the individual's engagement of the hypothalamic–pituitary–adrenal axis.'

The same happens when cold water swimming too, since according to the *Journal of Military Medicine*, 'Acclimatization to cold is a complicated phenomenon' but 'after repeated (5 to 10) exposures, less shivering is produced.[179] In fact, this adaptation can be so powerful that it's been reported nomadic civilisations of the arctic feel so comfortable in the cold they have no trouble sleeping in it.'[180]

THE WORLD'S STRONGEST ICE SWIMMER?

Back at Manley Mere and after 15 minutes Eddie emerged from the water, shivering but successful. Of course, we weren't safe yet. With his lips a strange shade of blue, it was clear the blood had drained from his skin and extremities (arms, legs, hands and feet) to increase blood flow to his core to protect his vital organs. As a result, I knew he was moments away from a severe case of 'after drop' and needed to re-heat his body as fast as possible. Fortunately, this wasn't my first rodeo and I had prepared a bag full of towels and thick woollen hats.

'Quick, put this on,' I said, passing him a knitted bobble hat.

'Ok, now what?' Eddie asked.

'We run and re-heat,' I said, sprinting in my trunks and woollen hat around the lake.

Understanding how important the next 15 minutes would be (and the severity of the 'after drop'), Eddie then burst into a sprint to catch me up. Aggressively generating heat through his giant quads, after just five minutes of running I then witnessed something I had never seen before. Eddie had an almost superhuman ability to re-heat and recover. When researching ice swimmers, scientists discovered subjects had a much higher percentage of body fat which can serve as a great way to insulate and retain heat.[181] Almost like a polar bear, seal and other cold-acclimatised animals.[182] Studies also found that muscle mass[183] helps to generate heat and Eddie had a plentiful amount of that too. It meant his 28 stone (177.8 kg) body possessed a unique amount of bulk (fat and muscle) to both generate heat and retain it.

In fact, by the time we finished a single loop of the lake (one mile) his lips were no longer a strange shade of blue and he was visibly sweating as steam could be seen from his gigantic shoulders as he stood there wearing nothing but a smile, swimming trunks and a bobble hat.

'What now?' he asked.

'We keep running,' I said.

We had now begun the Endurance-Based General Physical Preparedness part of the *Base Mesocycle* which would take place on the adventure trail that surrounded Manley Mere. Covered in thick mud that would tax the legs and the lungs, in many ways it was the perfect training ground to build an athletic base and 'get wintered' as we were forced to run, jump, climb and crawl around, through and over the woods.

ENDURANCE-BASED GENERAL PHYSICAL PREPAREDNESS

The Manley Mere adventure trail is 5 km (3.1 miles) long. Built back in 1994 by Kate's parents Mike and Jane, the entire family has always had a love for adventure and the great outdoors, so it only seemed logical for them to build an obstacle course to complement the water sports centre and sailing club they'd already converted from their dairy farm a decade before.

Densely populated with military-style tunnels, cargo nets and rope bridges, many of the zip lines and climbing frames were actually created for children and young teenagers, but in no way did this make them less valuable as a training tool based on the teachings of the PASM framework.

In fact, this was perfectly designed to help build kinaesthetic awareness. Don't be put off by the technical names. It's just a complex way of saying, 'Know where your body is in space.' Developing this ability gives you a better understanding of when the movements you're doing feel right or wrong. This kind of biological feedback helps you make adjustments to perform the movements better and more efficiently.

But before we even arrived at the first cargo net, Eddie wanted to voice some concerns.

'Ross, can I ask you a question?' he said.

'Sure, what's up?'

'Why are we still wearing our budgie smugglers while running barefoot through the woods? It feels like an odd way to spend the day training . . . can we not put some clothes on?' he asked, wondering what possible explanation I could give for the voluntary nudity.

'Well . . .' I said, pausing for a moment to consider how best to explain myself.

'I want us to train like Spartans.'

Eddie looked confused and told me he was unaware budgie smugglers formed part of the uniform of the feared and revered Spartan militia. But as we continued to run, I explained how our training today would take the teachings of the Russian Conjugate Sequence System and fuse it with the methodology of the Spartan bootcamp known as an *Agoge*.

Graduating from the Agoge was like a rite of passage for any young Spartan. Entering at the age of seven, they would be required to live and train among their peers in a culture where fierce (sometimes violent) competition was actively encouraged. At the age of twelve, young Spartans would graduate and be considered 'youths', at which point the Spartan training routine intensified with a stage of training that Eddie and I were currently practising.

Spartans would be required to run, train and live barefoot to toughen them up. But also, perhaps because they understood (on some level) the three inbuilt, primitive systems of biotensegrity, sensory feedback and the kinetic chain (discussed in the *Recovery*

Mesocycle chapter) that are positively influenced when barefoot running.

'That makes some sense,' Eddie conceded.

'But you still haven't told me why we're naked.'

Still running to our first obstacle, I then explained how young Spartans were given a single, thin cloak called a *Phoinikis* that they were expected to wear in any type of weather. It didn't matter come rain or shine, the purpose of wearing a Phoinikis was to (again) toughen them up psychologically and physiologically to extreme temperatures, from the bitter cold to stifling heat.

I could see Eddie was only semi-sold on my theory, but it didn't matter. Moments later (after 2 km of running and a Spartan history lesson) we'd arrived at a 20 ft high cargo net. Leading by example, I gripped the rope that was soaked and slippery from heavy rainfall days before and began my climb. But arriving at the top, the rope was then the least of my concerns. Now straddling the wooden beam at the summit of the structure, I was very aware my genitals were entirely unprotected from any rogue splinters that could be found in the rustic construction. Tentatively cupping my testicles, I shouted down to Eddie to warn him as he began his ascent,

'Quick word of warning, big man,' I said.

'Try to give the beam at the top a wide berth with your scrotum as you straddle it. I'm not sure our trunks offer much protection and that's a place no man wants to get a splinter.'

Obviously not thrilled to hear this, Eddie was also not one to back down from a challenge so continued to head for the peak, with his head held high and his penis tucked in.

By the time he reached the top, I had climbed down the other side and was safe, on the floor and with a splinter-less scrotum. But Eddie was now 20 ft in the air, in an incredibly precarious position with a leg either side of the cargo net.

'Now what?' he asked.

'Ok, commit and throw your back leg over the top like a round-house kick with enough clearance that you don't tear your testicles,' I said, but also very aware I was asking a 28 stone (177.8 kg) man to defy the laws of physics and physiology.

What I then witnessed was incredible.

It was like watching a rhino (known for its incredible strength) hanging from a tree like a monkey. It just didn't make sense that someone that size should have any degree of agility, yet there it was right before my eyes. In one fluid motion, Eddie performed a type of Kung Fu kick and then proceeded to front flip and climb down the other side of the cargo net with his genitals entirely intact.

The only explanation was that Eddie's childhood had followed the Russian Conjugate Sequence System, Process of Achieving Sports Mastery framework and was rooted in General Physical Preparedness. As a kid Eddie, excelled in many sports, but did *not* specialise. An elite-level national swimmer and gifted rugby player, he developed a well-rounded athletic base which improved his overall motor potential (neurological efficiency) and he didn't compete in England's Strongest Man competition until 2010 (aged 22) which he won despite entering at the last minute when a competitor dropped out due to injury.

Interestingly, this was also true of other great ancient Greek armies. This is why the Roman biographer Cornelius Nepos (110–25 BCE) wrote about famous Greek warriors undergoing training that focused on gymnastic ability and agility. When detailing the life of the celebrated Greek general of Thebes known as Epaminondas, Nepos wrote, 'After he grew up, and began to apply himself to gymnastic exercises, he studied not so much to increase the strength, as the agility, of his body; for he thought that strength suited the purposes of wrestlers, but that agility conduced to excellence in war. He used to exercise himself very much, therefore, in running and wrestling, as long as he could grapple, and contend standing, with his adversary.'[184]

Did it work? Well, worth noting is during the fourth century BCE it was Epaminondas who defeated the Spartan Army and transformed the Ancient Greek city-state of Thebes by revolutionising military training and tactics.

Essentially, history is riddled with examples of great humans achieving great things once they laid the foundation of a solid athletic base. Understand this and you begin to understand why Eddie (despite his gigantic frame) was able to sprint through streams, climb trees and hang from monkey bars. In fact, now 5 km into our run, it was clear no mud was too thick, no cargo net too high and no lake was too cold. He had conquered everything the Manley Mere adventure trail could throw at him.

That was until he met his arch nemesis.

You see, throughout history every superhero has had a weakness. For Superman it was kryptonite, but for Eddie his 'Achilles heel' came in a different form . . .

A 40 metre long tunnel.

Measuring just 1 metre in diameter, it was a 'snug' fit for myself. In fact, it was so narrow I couldn't actually crawl on my hands and knees and instead had to 'post' myself through the entrance on my belly and then (like a snake) inchworm my way through, one claustrophobic centimetre at a time. Requiring a lot of patience (and skin from my elbows, knees and stomach that grated along the floor) I made it to the other side and honestly thought Eddie wouldn't even attempt it. I was wrong. In the spirit of friendly competition inspired by the Spartan Agoge, he dived headfirst into the tunnel and followed my lead.

But after 10 metres he got stuck.

Unfortunately, the laws of geometry were never in Eddie's favour, and with the sheer size (and width) of his shoulders compared to the size of the tunnel, it was never going to end well.

'Ross, I think I'm stuck,' he said.

I paused to consider my response, because in all honesty I couldn't do a lot to help. My only other option would be to ring the fire brigade and ask them to free a 28 stone naked man from a tunnel on a kid's adventure trail. That's a phone call no-one wants to make. So instead, I tried coaching him towards the light.

'Ok, try to narrow your shoulders and rely less on your arms and elbows and instead propel yourself forward from the pelvis,' I replied.

'Got it,' he said, now making progress with his hips and humping the tunnel into submission.

'If you can get over halfway the tunnel becomes a little more slippery and lubricated from the rainwater and algae, so you can start to slide your way to freedom,' I said, trying to offer any words of encouragement that I could.

After what seemed like an eternity and through a strange, yet heroic display of athleticism, he finally emerged from the tunnel like a rhino giving birth. To this day, I'm not sure if Eddie moved through the tunnel or if the tunnel moved around him, but thanks to a weird and powerful form of 'pelvic propulsion' the man had managed to successfully defy the laws of geometry.

But with his sworn enemy slayed, our focus was now on clocking up some miles to train the heart, lungs and entire cardiorespiratory system to essentially 'build a bigger engine'. So, we headed into the woods (away from cargo nets and tunnels) and ran a steady 10 km.

BUILD A BIGGER ENGINE

Another focus of the *Base Mesocycle* is to train the cardiorespiratory system. This consists of the heart and blood vessels, which work with the respiratory system (the lungs and airways) to carry oxygen to the working muscles and organs during exercise and remove waste products like carbon dioxide during training. This is often what people are referring to when they say they want to 'build a bigger engine' or improve their 'gas tank'.

So, why is all this so important?

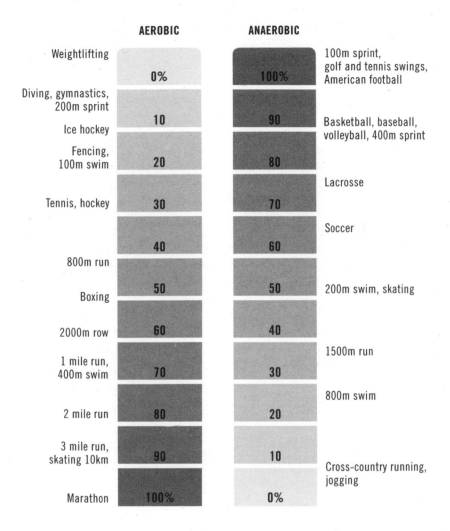

	AEROBIC	ANAEROBIC	
Weightlifting	0%	100%	100m sprint, golf and tennis swings, American football
Diving, gymnastics, 200m sprint	10	90	
Ice hockey			Basketball, baseball, volleyball, 400m sprint
Fencing, 100m swim	20	80	
			Lacrosse
Tennis, hockey	30	70	
	40	60	Soccer
800m run			
Boxing	50	50	200m swim, skating
2000m row	60	40	
1 mile run, 400m swim	70	30	1500m run
2 mile run	80	20	800m swim
3 mile run, skating 10km	90	10	
			Cross-country running, jogging
Marathon	100%	0%	

The main reason is because your heart and cardiorespiratory fitness are strongly related to your **aerobic energy system** which the body uses during low-intensity training that's *below* 70 per cent of your maximum effort, where the pace is slow and consistent (imagine the pace of a 40 km bike ride, a slow hike up a mountain or swimming 5 km downriver). Essentially, the body uses oxygen to create the molecular energy of the muscles needed to power all movements within the body (known as adenosine triphosphate) which means you can use this energy system for a long time to run, swim, hike or bike very far at a conservative pace. Put simply, the better your cardiorespiratory system the better your aerobic energy system and better physiologically equipped you are to run up mountains, swim downriver or row across oceans.

This is very different to your **anaerobic energy system**. This is what your body uses when the intensity of training is *above* 70 per cent of your maximum effort (imagine a two-minute fight or a 200-metre sprint across a frozen lake). Because the muscles are working at a pace that is too high to deliver oxygen to them, your body must break down carbohydrates from blood glucose or glucose stored in muscle to produce the molecular energy of the muscles needed to power all movements within the body.

All energy systems are constantly working at the same time. However, the predominant energy system used to re-supply adenosine triphosphate (molecular energy of the muscles) depends on the intensity and duration of the activity. In a graph, it looks like the figure on the previous page, where you will notice during most activities your energy systems are working together, you're just using different proportions/percentages of each.

Of course, most adventurers and athletes will have to operate over many different intensities and therefore will require an efficient aerobic and anaerobic energy system, but studies show the fitter you are (and the more efficient your cardiorespiratory system), the longer you can fuel your body with the aerobic system before the anaerobic system needs to take over.

The reason this is so important is because (as we know) the anaerobic energy system operates at *above* 70 per cent of your maximum effort, and since it cannot supply enough oxygen to the working muscles it must break down carbohydrates from blood glucose or glucose stored in muscle (muscle glycogen) to produce energy and 'power' the body. The problem is we only store a small amount of carbohydrates in the body, so the more we use the anaerobic energy system the faster we deplete this and then have to slow down or stop. As you can imagine, this would be terrible on an expedition if trekking through the Amazon rainforest or halfway up Everest.

This is why all athletes and adventurers need a solid aerobic base (made possible by a strong cardiorespiratory system) to support performance. One way to look at this is:

- Our **aerobic energy system** is our primary 'gas tank' which we rely on for a slow and steady speed in cruise control mode.
- Our **anaerobic energy system** is our 'jet engine afterburners' or nitrous oxide system (NOS) which we use to accelerate.

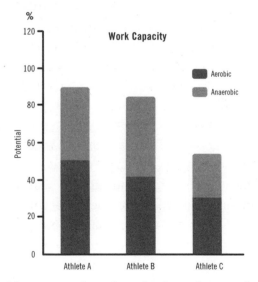

To use a working example, take a look at the graph above which shows three athletes:

- **Athlete A** has a strong aerobic energy system and an above-average anaerobic capacity.

- **Athlete B** has an above-average aerobic system but relies heavily on his superb anaerobic capacity.
- **Athlete C** is a relatively untrained, amateur athlete who is here for comparison.

While athletes A and B have a similar level of overall fitness, it's athlete A who has a stronger aerobic base, so during a long expedition (or event) they would be able to perform better as they would remain aerobic for longer before they have to tap into their anaerobic energy system. Note that both would perform on a similar level if the expedition (event) was short and intense, but over long distances it would be the superior aerobic system (gas tank) of athlete A that would be the determining factor of success.

So how do we do this?

The honest answer is, there's no exact blueprint for success. To demonstrate this, in a large-scale study conducted at the University of Hull, England researchers wanted to, 'Investigate whether there is currently sufficient scientific knowledge for scientists to be able to give valid training recommendations to long-distance runners and their coaches on how to most effectively enhance endurance.' What they concluded was, 'There is insufficient direct scientific evidence to formulate training recommendations based on the limited research. Although direct scientific evidence is limited, we believe that scientists can still formulate worthwhile training recommendations by integrating the information derived from training studies with other scientific knowledge.'[185]

This is exactly what Eddie and I were doing at Manley Mere. In a quest to build an aerobic base and bigger 'engine' we kept the volume high but intensity low based on the principles of *Zone Training*. This is a method of training where the pace and intensity of your workouts are determined by your heart rate, which is one of the best indicators of how hard your body is working during a workout. Put simply, we all have a personal resting heart rate (a minimum heart rate) and a maximum heart rate, but between these values are different heart rate zones that correspond to training intensity and training benefit. Now there are different ways to specify your heart rate zones, but one is to define them as percentages of your maximum heart rate, and that's what *Zone Training* focuses on.

Adopting a *Five-Zone Model of Endurance Training*, this is what your training 'zones' would look like when running, swimming, cycling or climbing:

Zone 1

- Working at 50–60 per cent of your maximum heart rate (aerobic in nature).
- You train in this zone during very low-intensity activities such as basic mobility work, a gentle walk, steady bike ride or very slow recovery run.

Zone 2

- Working at 60–70 per cent of your maximum heart rate (still aerobic).
- You train in this zone during low-intensity activities such as steady jog, brisk bike ride or a conservative swim pace. A good indicator of a Zone 2 activity is if you can hold a conversation and speak in complete sentences.

The difference between Zone 2 and Zone 3 is believed to be your anaerobic threshold.[186] This is the point when your body must switch from your aerobic energy system to your anaerobic energy system. The exact anaerobic threshold will vary from person to person and requires sophisticated laboratory techniques to measure it accurately,[187] but all athletes and adventures should at least be aware of this.

Zone 3

- Working at 70–80 per cent of your maximum heart rate.
- You train in this zone during a fast 10 km run or speedy 5 km swim as you begin to switch from your aerobic energy system to your anaerobic energy system.

Zone 4

- Working at 80–90 per cent of your maximum heart rate.
- You train in this zone during a very fast 1 km swim or fast ascent up an incredibly steep hill (you're now operating within the anaerobic realm).

Zone 5

- Working at 90–100 per cent of your maximum heart rate.
- This is essentially maximal effort (all-out sprint pace) and is very difficult to maintain for a prolonged time period.

So, that's the theory based on 'information derived from training studies with other scientific knowledge' (as recommended by the University of Hull).

Back at Manley Mere, what zone should and Eddie and I have been running in during our *Base Mesocycle*?

The answer was long, steady state sessions in Zone 2.

This is because studies show this can bring about many adaptations within the body that improve the cardiorespiratory system and build us a bigger 'gas tank'. One of the most well documented of these welcome adaptations is a stronger heart, since we've known for a long time that endurance training enables our hearts to grow bigger and stronger.[188] According to the *Olympic Textbook of Medicine in Sport* this was first described in 1899 when the Swedish physician

Salomon Henschen noted that cross-country skiers had larger hearts than the average person, a phenomenon thought to result from adaptation to long-term, intense aerobic exercise. After this initial discovery, more advanced imaging techniques were invented and we can now directly measure increases in the size and volume of our heart chambers (knowing our hearts are formed of four differently sized chambers). The top two chambers are called the **atria** and the bottom two are known as the **ventricles**.

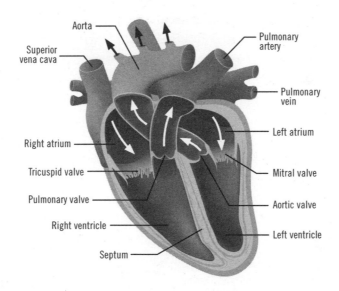

While all chambers need to function properly, the left ventricle is particularly important during exercise as it pumps freshly oxygenated blood to supply our working muscles. Indeed, studies suggest that the size and volume of the left ventricle increases in response to exercise. In fact, one study published in the *Journal of the American College of Cardiology* found that three years of professional cycling led to a 2 mm increase in left ventricular diameter (the distance between opposing walls of the left ventricle) from 58.3 mm to 60.3 mm.[189]

Another study found that exercise in previously untrained people resulted in an increase in the volume of both right and left ventricles at the end of diastole (the phase of the heartbeat when the heart muscle relaxes and allows the ventricles to fill with blood).[190] This is obviously a welcome adaptation, since it allows more blood (and oxygen) to be pumped with each heartbeat. In physiological terms, we say the heart has a higher stroke volume, and the greater this is the more blood and oxygen can be delivered to the working muscles.

Another benefit of endurance training is the heart not only increases in size, it also increases in thickness as there's an increase in size of individual heart muscle cells (myocytes) that thickens the walls of our heart chambers and allows the heart to contract more forcefully and pump harder.

These two adaptations combined can result in a lower resting heart rate since larger and more powerful hearts are capable of pumping a greater volume of blood with each beat, which in turn means they do not need to beat as fast to sustain an adequate output of blood to tissues and organs at rest. How low? Well, the five-time Tour de France winner Miguel Indurain had a resting heart rate of just 28 beats per minute, which means it's fair to say he had a pretty sizeable 'gas tank'.

Finally, other welcome adaptations for endurance are:[191]

- An increased mitochondria density.[192] These are often called the powerhouses of cells and play a vital role in the conversion of energy from food, so having more of them results in more efficient energy production and oxygen transportation, allowing you to sustain a higher percentage of your aerobic capacity.
- Increased blood plasma volume[193] which helps increase stroke volume and therefore the amount of oxygen your body can use during exercise.[194]
- Aerobic training can also bring your body into a more parasympathetic state[195] compared to high-intensity training,

decreasing your sympathetic drive and allowing you to rest and recover more effectively (very important during the early stages of the *Base Mesocycle* when you consider you've only just finished the *Recovery Mesocycle.*)

And what's more, sports science is still uncovering other adaptations.

But here's an important point to consider: this doesn't mean Eddie and I should spend the entire year training in Zone 2, running around the woods in our budgie smugglers at a slow and steady pace and neglecting any form of high-intensity (anaerobic) training in Zones 3, 4 and 5. No, when looking at the year's training plan in its entirety (the complete periodised macrocycle) you will notice the:

- **Base Mesocycle** operates within the aerobic realm (Zone 2) where volume is high and intensity is low.

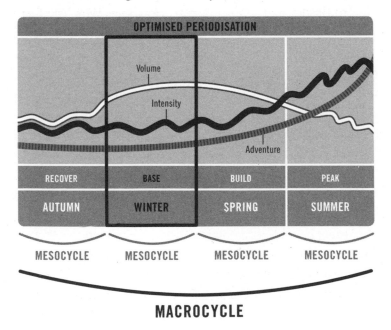

This then lays the 'foundations' for the:

- **Build Mesocycle** that begins to train the anaerobic energy system more as the intensity is high and volume is decreased.

By adopting this holistic approach to training the body through the year, you understand how each mesocycle works in synergy to (jointly) improve your body's ability to use both the aerobic energy system (at low intensity) and anaerobic energy system (at high intensity) to provide enough energy to continue to operate whatever the pace of the hike, run or cycle.

So after another few laps of the trail, we clocked 15 km in total and decided our endurance-based (Spartan and Soviet-inspired) General Physical Preparedness was done and our 'gas tanks' were sufficiently trained for the day. So, we scaled our final cargo net and headed to the farmyard to begin strongman training.

STRENGTH-BASED GENERAL PHYSICAL PREPAREDNESS

The time was 4 p.m. and the sun was fading fast as the evening approached. We had been swimming across lakes, climbing over obstacles and crawling through tunnels for nearly six hours. Cold, wet, hungry and still (semi) naked in our trunks, it's hard to know exactly how many calories we'd burned that day. Studies have shown that whether you're running, cycling or crawling, the heavier you are the more calories you burn. According to scientists from Israel's Chaim Sheba Medical Center,[196] the additional weight alters your 'locomotion biomechanics' – basically your technique – which leads to a 'Significant increase in energy (calorie) cost over time.'

Couple this with the fact that Eddie and I were attacking an adventure trail in the British winter wearing nothing but a Spartan-inspired 'banana hammock' (research shows shivering can burn up to 425 calories per hour[197] and brings about biochemical changes[198] that send your energy expenditure[199] through the roof[200]) and it's clear the calorie requirements for his 28 stone (177.8 kg) frame and my 16 stone (101 kg) sea-bulked body would be elevated far beyond a conventional and gentle 24 km run.

But this was good and these conditions were ideal.

When training for an expedition (on land or sea) there *needs* to be a distinction between training as an athlete and training as an adventurer. This is so important. Relating back to the concept of *Stoic Sports Science* (that I introduced in my book *The Art of Resilience*) where I needed a philosophy to mentally cope under adverse conditions that were outside of the realms of conventional sport, the same must be true when training for an adventure as well.

Put simply, great adventurers do not necessarily make great athletes and great athletes do not necessarily make great adventurers, since the conditions and demands on the body and mind are entirely different and this must be reflected in the training.

Neither is better or worse, just different.

For instance, remember when earlier we talked about Eliud Kipchoge becoming the first human to run a marathon in under two hours? To achieve this, the conditions of his training were closely controlled down to the finest detail to replicate race day, as temperature, weather, gradient, pacing and even wind resistance were all manipulated to allow for optimal conditions. In contrast, on 29 May 1953, Edmund Hillary and Tenzing Norgay summited Everest where the conditions were wildly uncontrollable compared to Kipchoge's physical endeavour.

Of course, both were incredible pioneering feats that advanced our understanding of the human body. But a key difference is adventurers must train under harsh, unpredictable conditions and your *Base Mesocycle* is the ideal time to begin trialling this. I call it *Adversity Training* and it is essentially Soviet-inspired General Physical Preparedness under Spartan-like conditions. You're running, climbing, swimming, crawling, pushing, pulling, lifting and throwing while often hungry, cold and fatigued. Technique is often ugly and conditions are rarely pleasant.

This is why trainee Spartans would only be given a small amount of food each day despite brutal training regimes that were high in volume such as a long march. The aim was to keep them lean, light, hungry and motivated. In fact, if they wanted/needed more food they were encouraged to steal, since this taught them to be resourceful and cunning, but if they were caught they were brutally punished. Not for stealing, but for not stealing well enough.

In fact, Spartans rarely ate for pleasure and it was more a means of survival. Need proof? A staple of their diet was *melas zomos* (black broth) made from boiled pigs' legs, blood, salt and vinegar. According to legend, a man from Sybaris, a city in southern Italy infamous for its luxury and gluttony, after tasting the Spartans' black soup remarked with disgust, 'Now I do perceive why it is that Spartan soldiers encounter death so joyfully; dead men require no longer to eat; black broth is no longer a necessity.'[201]

Basically, even a Spartan's tastebuds were hard and durable. According to Aristotle this coupled with 'laborious exercises' all served to 'make their boys animal in nature' and contribute to 'manly courage'.[202] This is why it's been said for Spartans, going into battle was relatively more comfortable than their Spartan training.

Other famous Greek military leaders were also keen to make a distinction between their sportsmen and soldiers. It is well documented that the celebrated Greek general and statesman Philopoemen (253–183 BCE) believed that the diet and training regime of an athlete should be highly strict and consistent, but in contrast a warrior needed to be able to survive on little food and endure extreme sleep deprivation.

In the book *War and Games* by Tim Cornell, it states Philopoemen even banned sport and athletics for his soldiers, believing, 'The habit of body and mode of life for athlete and soldier were totally different, and particularly that their diet and training were not the same, since the one required much sleep, continuous surfeit of food, and fixed periods of activity and repose, in order to preserve or improve their condition, which the slightest influence or the least departure from routine is apt to change for the worse; whereas the soldier ought to be conversant with all sorts of irregularity and all sorts of inequality, and above all should accustom himself to endure lack of food easily, and as easily lack of sleep.'[203]

Did it work? Well, Philopoemen and his military methodology was famous for defeating the Spartan Army in 222 BCE in the Battle of Sellasia and he was appointed as *Strategos* (military general) on eight occasions. So yes, I would say he was right to make the important distinction between being a solider and being an athlete.

Of course, I am not (and likely neither are you) an ancient Greek warrior.

Which is why (again) the *Base Mesocycle* takes inspiration from sportsmen of the Soviet Union system and soldiers of the Ancient Greek Army and is also why, back in Manley Mere, Eddie and I decided to forgo rest, recovery and food and instead take a tractor for a 5 km run as we pushed it around the farmyard to build *Work Capacity*.

The most underrated component for many athletes, but an absolute necessity for adventurers on expeditions that can take place over days, weeks or months, work capacity is essentially the total amount of training you can perform, recover from and adapt positively to.

For athletes in training, a high work capacity means:

- You can train harder and for longer.
- You are less prone to overtraining.

For adventurers during an expedition, a high work capacity means:

- You can continue to progress day after day.
- You can function on less rest and recovery.

This last point is interesting, since during extreme expeditions the body is essentially breaking down as your level of physical exertion far surpasses your rate of recovery. This is sometimes unavoidable and so while it can't be stopped, the goal of any adventurer should be to delay or slow this inevitable degradation of the body (and brain).

One great example of this is the Talisker Whisky Atlantic Challenge, a 3,000-mile row from the Canary Islands to Antigua. Every year, the fleet of competitors contains groups of elite-level rowers with beautiful biomechanics, power, speed and stamina who race to become the first to make the historic ocean crossing. But so often it's not the best rowers that win. No, it's those with the highest work capacity. Those with an ability to recover from 60-plus miles of rowing per day, on very little sleep and recovery, for over a month as the body and brain begins to degrade. This is no exaggeration either, since I've had many friends complete the row and while the media publish many articles about the heroics of these incredible men and women who make the voyage, I've been privy to many conversations about the body and brain breaking down that weren't quite fit for public broadcast. Stories that two friends of mine kindly granted me permission to share with you now:

CHARLIE PITCHER

Charlie is one of the world's most experienced ocean rowers and has been a professional international yachtsman for over 20 years. What's more, he's an accomplished ultra-runner and competed in the Marathon des Sables in 2009 and undertook a gruelling 350-mile charity trail run across Scotland in just four days in 2011. All things considered, he has an incredible work capacity.

In 2013, he used this to break the solo Atlantic rowing record, making the 3,000-mile journey in 35 days. But what the records books don't show is he had to row through complete exhaustion under the blazing sun and suffered from severe hallucinations for days in the process. Speaking to him after his voyage, I asked him what he saw. His reply was one I was not expecting.

'Well, I'd been at sea 27 days,' he said. 'I was only a few hundred miles away from land and knew the record was within my grasp, but there was a slight problem.'

He paused to consider the best way to explain his dilemma to me.

'Storm? Shark? Hole in the boat?' I asked.

'No, no, nothing like that,' he said.

'Then what?' I asked, now confused.

'It was the mermaid sitting on the hull of my rowing boat,' he said with a completely straight face.

'She'd been there for a few days and while I did appreciate the company, I was conscious I needed to really crack on if I was to beat the record so I had to ask her to leave,' he said, still deadly serious.

'And?' I asked.

'Well, as you can imagine she wasn't happy. She jumped off the boat and whipped her tail, splashing me in the process, but I told her I didn't have a choice and needed to break the record,' he said with a genuine look of disappointment on his face.

At the time, I didn't know whether to laugh or console my friend. But putting Charlie's broken friendship with his beloved mermaid companion to one side, this remains one of the best examples of the body's ability to continue despite the brain breaking down when you're equipped with a large enough work capacity and a complete refusal to quit.

JASON FOX

Jason is a former Royal Marine Commando and was a Special Forces Sergeant for over 20 years. Built like a tank, it's also fair to say he has the work capacity of a thoroughbred horse, which explains why in 2016 he (and four friends) were able to set the record for the fastest, unsupported crew to row the longest route across the Atlantic Ocean. Rowing 3,308 nautical miles from Portugal to Venezuela in just 50 days, they capsized three times, endured storms, 20 ft waves and were stalked by a shark for miles. But when I asked him about the worst part, his answer was one that still haunts my rowing workouts to this day.

'It was an injury none of us expected,' he said.

Intrigued, I urged him to go on.

'You know people can develop pressure sores and ulcers on areas of the skin that are under pressure from lying in bed, sitting in a wheelchair or wearing a cast for a prolonged period of time?' he asked.

'Yes,' I said, familiar with it but unsure how it related to his row.

'Well, it can be made much worse when rowing across an ocean since you're sat in one position for hours, days and weeks with your hands practically glued and grasped to the oars as the waves crash over the boat and soak your clothes, and the saltwater can make these ulcers so much worse,' he said.

'So, your hands took a battering?' I replied.

'Not my hands,' he said. 'A month in, I developed a BIG boil (ulcer) on my hoop.'

By 'hoop' he was referring to his bum hole and yes, this story still haunts any lengthy workout I ever do on an indoor rowing machine. But unable to shake this story from my memory, I was curious how he continued all the way to Venezuela while nursing an injury that was so hard to treat.

'You know the cushions that are shaped like a hoop that people sit on when they have piles to protect their delicate bum hole?' he said.

'Yes,' I replied, vaguely aware of the concept.

'Well, we learnt to make a homemade version from a rolled-up t-shirt that we wrapped in silver tape. We called it the "space pretzel" but the problem was everyone began suffering from similar ulcers in similar places, which meant our new invention got used a lot and would then lose its shape as everyone shared the communal space pretzel.'

'So, when rowing across oceans you basically need a bespoke space pretzel unique for your bum hole only?' I asked.

'Yes, basically,' he said smiling as if recalling fond memories of the sea and his beloved space pretzel.

To this day this brutal (bum-hole) story remains one of the best examples of the brain's ability to continue despite the body breaking down when you're equipped with a large enough work capacity, and I'll forever be grateful to Jason sharing it with the world.

HOMEGROWN HORSEPOWER (WORK CAPACITY)

Back in Manley Mere (and long before I embarked on another adventure), I was determined to rebuild my own work capacity. How? There are many ways, but the slow and strategic accumulation of hours of high-volume and low-intensity General Physical Preparedness (both endurance and strength based) within the *Base Mesocycle* is ideal.

Eddie and I weren't struggling and straining when pushing the tractor since the goal wasn't to improve strength (the body's ability to generate force). Nor was it to enhance speed (the quickness of movement of a limb) or cardiorespiratory endurance (the prolonged ability of the heart and lungs to supply muscles with nutrients and oxygen). Instead, it was to 'train the body to train' and (again) build an 'athletic base' to tolerate harder, heavier or more intense sessions later when beginning the *Build Mesocycle*. All of which was done by calculating the work capacity of that session.

THE MATHS: MEASURING WORK CAPACITY

Low-intensity General Physical Preparedness requires both strength, muscular endurance and cardiorespiratory endurance. While there are various methods used to test each, some of the most common techniques are as follows:

- **Strength.** Can be tested by measuring someone's 1RM on a particular lift (this is the maximum weight a person can squat, bench or deadlift once).
- **Muscular Endurance.** Can be tested on a specific muscle group by seeing how many repetitions someone can complete in a minute.
- **Cardiorespiratory Endurance.** Can be measured through VO2 max testing. VO2 max is essentially a measurement of the maximum amount of oxygen that your body is capable of consuming to generate energy that can be used at the cellular level (the 'gold standard' of VO2 max testing requires laboratory conditions).

But it's somewhere between these three standards that we will find work capacity.

Touching upon various physiological variables, one way of calculating this is by measuring 'power' based on its physical and biomechanical definition:

Power (P) = Work (w)/Time (t)

'Power' is defined (within strength and conditioning) as the rate of doing work which is measured in Watts (W). For those interested in the equations take a look at the following (but if not, don't worry, just skip ahead):

Power (P) = Work (w)/Time (t)
Work (w) = Force (f) x Displacement (d)
Force (f) = Acceleration (a) x Mass (m)
Acceleration (a) = ΔVelocity (Δv)/Time (t)
Velocity (v) = Displacement (d)/Time (t)
Thus . . .
Power (P) = Mass (m) x Displacement[200] (d2)/Time[201] (t3)

Again, if you don't like maths, no problem. What matters is you understand that power relies on three things, and to increase power (work capacity) during training, you must alter one of these three things by:

- Moving heavier stuff (increase mass).
- Moving stuff further (increase displacement).
- Moving stuff faster (decrease time).

Improving any one of these factors (even while the other two remain the same) will have a positive effect on power. So around the farmyard at Manley Mere, Eddie and I chose to 'move stuff further' and increase displacement as we pushed the tractor for 5 km in total.

As we did, I told Eddie about the adventurer awards ceremony back in December and my subsequent desire to avoid 'spiritual decay' and my innate desire for adventure again.

'I understand,' Eddie said. 'At the 2016 World Deadlift Championship I made history and deadlifted 500 kg (1,102 lb) and a year later won World's Strongest Man. It would have been so easy for me to retire, since I had achieved everything I ever wanted.'

I nodded. It was true. All before the age of 30, Eddie had nothing left to prove or achieve, but for reasons related to askēsis and eustress, here he was pushing a tractor around a farmyard in pursuit of some form of eudaimonia.

BLUEPRINT

'Can I ask you something?' Eddie asked.

'Sure,' I replied.

'Do you think Aristotle ever pushed a tractor in his pants to develop "manly courage", or Philopoemen ever got stuck in a tunnel looking for eudaimonia?'

'Maybe,' I said. 'They probably just left that out of the books they published.'

As the sun began to set in the sky, we continued to push the tractor while talking about the philosophy of fitness and adventure, all to civilise the mind and savage the body as we rebuilt my athletic base.

BASE TRAINING PLAN (WINTER): MICROCYCLE (WEEK'S PLAN)

The strength workouts themselves are (again) biomechanically divided. This is mainly to keep the workouts simple throughout the entire macrocycle, since 'push', 'pull' and 'lower body' movements are easy to follow and encourage big, functional movements that use universal motor recruitment patterns that continue to help develop neurological efficiency.

As the volume of this mesocycle increases (but intensity remains low) the microcycle contains EIGHT sessions per week which consists of:

- THREE strength sessions that continue to develop the strength-based rehab practised during the *Recovery Mesocycle* to rebuild the durability of the muscles, ligaments and tendons.
- FOUR (low-intensity) Endurance-Based General Physical Preparedness operating in Zone 2 to build a solid aerobic base ('gas tank').
- ONE Strongman strength session rooted in General Physical Preparedness to improve work capacity and the body's ability to handle more training.

Finally, within this mesocycle the scheduling of the sessions is so important. This is because during your *Base Mesocycle* you begin to perform two sessions per day, so (at first as your body adapts to this new work capacity) your recovery will be on a 'knife edge', meaning when there is no training session planned you must continue to consciously activate your parasympathetic nervous system and continue to prioritise sleep.

But the other reason it's so important to schedule (and separate) your workouts is because during each session you're trying to elicit a different physiological adaptation within the body, whether that's improving strength in the gym or aerobic fitness during a trail run. This can become complicated in your conditioning, as research published in 1980 in the *European Journal of Applied Physiology and Occupational Physiology* found that if your strength and stamina workouts are too close together (without enough recovery in between) you can 'dilute' the effectiveness of your training and won't improve optimally in one area.

Why? Because your body doesn't know whether to become stronger or more endured as the 'potency' of your training stimulus is lost. Studies at the Division of Molecular Physiology at Dundee University found that strength training and endurance training bring about very different adaptations within the body, and combining both 'blocks each other's signalling' to adapt. They stated, 'During the last several decades many researchers have reported an interference effect when strength and endurance were trained concurrently (together).'[204]

Known as the 'interference phenomenon', studies show your body doesn't know whether it's adapting to strength or stamina and so doesn't optimally adapt to either. But when you consider your macrocycle within its entirety, you understand it is possible to send a clear 'cellular signal' to the body to adapt to multiple workouts in a single day:

- If you separate your workouts enough within a 24-hour period.
- Plan your training effectively within a microcycle (a week).
- If you improve your work capacity enough (during the *Base Mesocycle*).

In summary, the focus of this entire mesocycle is to build an athletic base by training to train. This is all in preparation for the harder, heavier and more intense sessions that will follow during the *Build Mesocycle*. Represented in a table, a week's training looks like this:

	Monday	Tuesday	Wednesday	Thursday	Friday	Saturday	Sunday
MORNING	Swim 5–10 km Open water	'Pull' Routine	Leg Routine	'Push' Routine	Weighted Run	General Physical Preparedness	Rest
PURPOSE	Aerobic Fitness (Zone 2) and Work Capacity	(Continued) Strength-Based Prehab/Rehab	(Continued) Strength-Based Prehab/Rehab	(Continued) Strength-Based Prehab/Rehab	Aerobic Fitness (Zone 2) and Work Capacity	(Continued) Strength-Based Prehab/Rehab and Work Capacity	Rest
AFTERNOON		Weighted Run		Swim 5–10 km Open water			
PURPOSE		Aerobic Fitness (Zone 2) and Work Capacity		Aerobic Fitness (Zone 2) and Work Capacity			Rest

6-DAY BASE PROGRAMME
MONDAY & FRIDAY
ENDURANCE-BASED GENERAL PHYSICAL PREPAREDNESS

LOW-INTENSITY STEADY STATE SWIM: WORK CAPACITY

Exercises	Time	Distance	Intensity
Swim	60+ minutes	Irrelevant	Zone 2 60–70 per cent of your maximum heart rate

Coaching Cues

As mentioned previously, the National Strength and Conditioning Association believes long-slow distance running or swimming is a great way to 'increase the athlete's tolerance for more intense training'. This is why even if your goal isn't to be an open water swimmer, as a training 'tool' (during your Base Mesocycle) swimming is brilliant as it's a non-weight bearing exercise, which allows you to train work capacity while still continuing to care for the joints, muscles and tendons post-Recovery Mesocycle.

ENDURANCE-BASED GENERAL PHYSICAL PREPAREDNESS
(WORK CAPACITY) WEIGHTED RUNS: WORK CAPACITY

Exercises	Time	Distance	Intensity
Run	60+ minutes	Irrelevant	Zone 2 60–70 per cent of your maximum heart rate

Coaching Cues

The goal is to continue barefoot running rehab, but begin to fuse it with principles of General Physical Preparedness to improve work capacity. This is why the runs are performed weighted, since (as previously mentioned) to improve work capacity/power you must:

- Move heavier stuff (increase mass).
- Move stuff further (increase displacement).
- Move stuff faster (decrease time).

Although a prowler push/sled drag is ideal (or even pushing a tractor), if you don't have access to these, adding weight to your runs allows you to improve work capacity through endurance-based general physical preparedness.

TUESDAY: 'PULL' TRAINING

Exercises	Repetitions	Sets	Rest	Physiological Adaptation
Passive Hang (Brachiating) (p 301)	30–45 seconds	3	90 seconds	Strength Rehab/ Prehab
Scapula Pull-Ups (p 302)	10	3	90 seconds	Strength Rehab/ Prehab
Overhand (p 303) (pronated) Pull-Ups (Optional: Weighted)	8–10	3	90 seconds	Strength-Based Work Capacity
Underhand (supinated) Close-Grip Pull-Ups (p 304) (Optional: Weighted)	8–10	3	90 seconds	Strength-Based Work Capacity
Single-Arm Dumbbell Row (p 304)	10 (each arm)	3	60 seconds	Strength-Based Work Capacity
Spider Bicep Curls (p 305)	10	3	60 seconds	Strength-Based Work Capacity
Rope Pulls (p 305)	20 metres	3	45 seconds	Strength-Based Work Capacity

WEDNESDAY: LEG ROUTINE

Exercises	Repetitions	Sets	Rest	Physiological Adaptation
Seated (box) Squats (p 312)	8–10	3	90 seconds	Strength-Based Work Capacity
(Barbell) Reverse Lunges (p 314)	10 metres (backward)	4	60 seconds	Strength-Based Work Capacity
Single-Arm Overhead Kettlebell Lunge (p 314)	10 (each leg)	4	60 seconds	Strength-Based Work Capacity
Barbell Standing Barefoot Calf (Toe) Raises (p 313)	10	3	90 seconds	Strength-Based Work Capacity
Prowler Push (p 315)	40 metres (if limited space, perform 20 metres back and forth for one round)	5	45 seconds	Strength-Based Work Capacity

THURSDAY: 'PUSH' TRAINING

Exercises	Repetitions	Sets	Rest	Physiological Adaptation
Scapula Push-Ups (p 319)	10	3	90 seconds	Strength Rehab/Prehab
Barbell Bench Press (p 322)	8–10	3	90 seconds	Strength-Based Work Capacity
Standing Barbell Shoulder Press (p 324)	8–10	3	90 seconds	Strength-Based Work Capacity
Ring Dips (p 324)	8–10	3	90 seconds	Strength-Based Work Capacity
Tricep Pushdowns (p 323)	12	3	60 seconds	Strength-Based Work Capacity
Bear Crawls (p 325)	10 metres forward then 10 metres back	3	45 seconds	Strength-Based Work Capacity

SATURDAY: 'STRONGMAN' SESSION

Exercises	Repetitions	Sets	Rest	Physiological Adaptation
Sledge Hammers (p 327)	20	5	45 seconds	Strength-Based Work Capacity and Strongman General Physical Preparedness
Tyre Flips (p 328)	20	5	45 seconds	Strength-Based Work Capacity and Strongman General Physical Preparedness
Bear hug Carry (p 329)	10 metres forward then 10 metres back	5	45 seconds	Strength-Based Work Capacity and Strongman General Physical Preparedness
Plate Pinch Farmers Walk (p 329)	10 metres forward then 10 metres back	3	45 seconds	Strength-Based Work Capacity and Strongman General Physical Preparedness

SPRING | BUILD MESOCYCLE OVERVIEW

'CIVILISE THE MIND, BUT MAKE SAVAGE THE BODY'

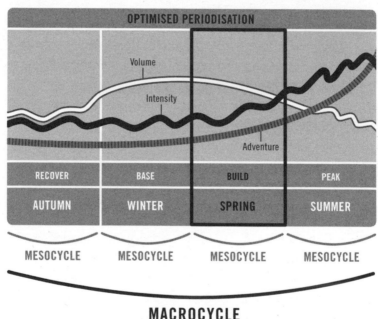

After a hard winter's training my *Base Mesocycle* was complete. As a result, I had built a strong athletic foundation (work capacity) through Soviet–Spartan-inspired training and now my body could tolerate longer, harder and heavier training sessions. Throughout the spring, I would begin my *Build Mesocycle* and my goals would become focused on:

- **Developing *Specific* Physical Preparedness (SPP).** This is based on the teachings of the Russian Conjugate Sequence System and Process of Achieving Sports Mastery (of the 1960s and early 1970s). Since now I had developed General Physical Preparedness through the *Base Mesocycle,* I was ready to make my training more specific to sea swimming through Specific Physical Preparedness.
- **Train Strength through the Force-Velocity Curve.** Most sports and adventurers require different forms of strength, which is why we must move from functional strength developed through work capacity, to explosive power and speed with a greater intensity generating greater force (Force = Mass x Acceleration). The entire time training the specific strength-speed qualities of your particular sport.
- **Increasing High-Intensity (Anaerobic) Fitness.** Improving on the aerobic base ('gas tank') built during the *Build Mesocycle* when training at low intensities for long periods (Zone 2), the goal is to condition the body to work more efficiently at high intensities (improving our 'jet engine afterburners').
- **Train Pain Tolerance.** As the intensity of training increases (and volume decreases), I had to recalibrate my perception to pain. This is because although I was now physically ready to tolerate harder sessions, I had to ensure I was mentally equipped to do so too.

In summary, your *Build Mesocycle* is the time to specialise in your chosen sport. As mentioned before, during the initial General Physical Preparedness stage (your *Base Mesocycle*) the amount of sport-specific exercise is limited and constitutes only 5–10 per cent of the total training volume to avoid specialising too early. But after developing a well-rounded athletic base, your overall motor potential would have improved which means you can specialise in a sport with newly developed neurological efficiency and the ability to tolerate longer, harder and heavier training sessions. This means if you want to begin training to hit a personal best for a marathon or maybe attack your first triathlon, now is the time to start, safe in the knowledge you have a bulletproof body that's been built on rock-solid foundations (see the 18-Week Marathon Guide and 12-Week Triathlon Guide at the end of this chapter). But understand now you're better equipped to specialise in anything. For me (in 2019) this meant trying to use my newly formed athletic base to try and survive on a grappling mat with one of the world's greatest martial artists.

STARTING MY BUILD MESOCYCLE
SPRING 2019, NOTTINGHAM, ENGLAND

It was 10 March 2019 and I had arrived at the entrance to the gym. My mood was best described as clueless, yet keen. For although I'd dabbled in boxing and wrestling before (and was a huge fan of those sports), I could count on two hands the hours of martial arts training that I had. Basically, if there was a grade lower than a white belt, that would be me.

But despite being nervous and utterly out of my depth, my lack of skill didn't matter since my goal wasn't to become a black belt in Brazilian jiu-jitsu or make my professional boxing debut. No, my goal was to train pain tolerance and, to quote the Roman emperor and philosopher Marcus Aurelius, 'Wrestle to be the man philosophy wished to make you.'

I love this quote since the sentiment was shared by Plato too. A renowned philosopher but also an accomplished wrestler and gymnast, he competed at the Isthmian Games (comparable to the Olympics) and his actual name was Aristocles, but 'Plato' was given to him by his wrestling coach because of his broad shoulders (in Greek, *Platon* means 'broad'). In his (last and longest) work entitled *Laws*, he celebrated the benefits of stand-up grappling claiming it had military use, developing 'strength and health' for the battlefield. But it also cultivated character if 'practised with a gallant spirit', since it was believed physical virtues encourage psychological excellence in the form of perseverance and courage.

According to research, his teacher Socrates agreed too and it's believed they actually met in a wrestling gymnasium during the fifth century BCE.[205] This would have been quite common since gymnasiums were popular hangouts for young men in Athens and other Hellenic cities during this time, as they functioned as a training facility for competitors in public games such as wrestling, but were also places for socialising and engaging in intellectual pursuits.

For this visit to my friend's gym in Nottingham, and despite being wildly unqualified, I was warmly welcomed through the doors and was told I was in safe hands during my maiden voyage into mixed martial arts. Why? Because the aforementioned friend and gym owner was Dan Hardy. One of the greatest mixed martial artists to have ever walked the earth, having claimed numerous championship belts at welterweight, Dan was now a coach and one of the world's most respected analytical experts on modern combat sports.

But as a student that day, I did have one thing in my favour . . . a good *Base Mesocycle*. What I lacked in skill I made up for in a developed neurological efficiency to improve and high work capacity to positively adapt to the hours of training needed to learn. I was basically a malleable ball of clay that Dan could spar, strike and submit, which he did with ease but ever so politely. In fact, on one occasion he even threw me over his shoulder (when demonstrating judo throws) but took particular care mid-throw to cradle my head and place me gently on the canvas as I hit the floor.

'You ok, buddy?' he asked as he helped me up from the mat.

'Yes. I've never been so politely beaten up before,' I replied laughing.

Dan smiled, almost apologetic about his superior combat skills and strength. But with some technique now taught, he then invited me to sit on the mat as he explained how mixed martial arts had evolved so much through the years, so I could better understand the methodology of today's training session and why my body and ego would take such a beating for the next few hours.

'Our sport dates back to the Greek Olympic Games in 648 BCE,' he began, 'in an event called Pankration [meaning 'all force']. It fused boxing and wrestling techniques along with holds, kicks and chokes.'

Sitting cross-legged on the mat, I loved ancient Greek history so urged Dan to go on.

'It's a sport wrapped in mystic and mythology and legend has it that Hercules developed Pankration in order to dominate in wrestling tournaments and Theseus used it to defeat the Minotaur. Of course, these are just myths, but the fact that Pankration is connected to these respected heroes shows its importance to Ancient Greek culture.'

Needless to say, I was immediately a fan of any sport that contained stories of mythical half-man, half-bull beasts so began asking about the rules.

'There weren't many,' he said. 'One ancient account tells of a situation in which the judges were trying to determine the winner of a match. The difficulty lay in that fact that both men had died in the arena from their injuries, making it hard to determine a victor. Eventually, the judges decided the winner was the one who didn't have his eyes gouged out.' Dan seemed quite unaffected by the brutality of his story.

As for me, visibly wincing, I was less desensitised to this level of violence. But this is why Dan was a different breed of human. I called him a 'savage scholar' since he studied the history, philosophy and science of fighting all his life, so when describing Pankration eye-gouging techniques, it was like he was describing a cricket match or a friendly game of golf.

MIXED MARTIAL ARTS AND MILITARY TRAINING: TRAIN THE PAIN

If you understand the science[206] [207] of pain tolerance,[208] [209] you begin to understand the chivalry and savagery of Dan Hardy and how the world's most elite fighters have scientifically and strategically re-wired their own brains. In fact, modern research has shown, 'Martial arts athletes have a different sensitivity to pain compared to non-athletes,' likely due to the 'systematic exposure to brief periods of intense pain during training or competition'.[210]

Sitting on the grappling mats that day, I asked Dan what forms of 'systematic exposure to brief periods of intense pain' he'd studied through his 20-year career. He then told me six methods of fighting and training, from martial arts and the military, that I will never forget and will likely never try.

1. Muay Thai Shin Conditioning

Muay Thai is a combat sport of Thailand known as the 'art of eight limbs' since athletes will use their fists, elbows, knees and shins to strike their opponent. This is why Muay Thai fighters will go to extreme lengths to toughen up these parts of the body. One method that is still widely used today is kicking a banana tree (repeatedly) with the shins. Interestingly, the adaptation to training here isn't just mental, it's physical too. That's because this method of conditioning causes microfractures in the bone and, through a process known as ossification, the fractured bones are repaired and become denser and stronger due to the new bone tissue created.

2. Spetsnaz Smashing Bricks

Russia is a country renowned for its military prowess, but it's specifically the special-purpose military units known as Spetsnaz that are considered among the toughest and most durable in the world. That's because if conducting basic training in sub-zero Arctic conditions wasn't enough, they also practise building up their tolerance to pain by smashing massive cinder blocks on each other with giant sledge hammers.

3. North Korean 'Iron Fists'

Perhaps the most secretive (almost mythical) method of training on this list belongs to the North Korean Storm Corps. Believed to undergo some of the most brutal training in the world, according to an alleged defector, recruits are required to punch a tree trunk 5,000 times in a row, then punch a jagged tin can until their hand is completely bloodied, before punching a pile of salt. No doubt applying a similar methodology to Muay Thai fighters, the theory is to turn the hands into rock-hard weapons.

4. Tameshiwari: The 'Art of Breaking Stuff'

Tameshiwari really is just the art of smashing and breaking things with your hands, feet, head and elbows. Popularised by the founder of Japanese Kyokushin karate, Masutatsu Oyama, tameshiwari practitioners will break wood, bricks, stone and even ice with parts of their body to measure the force of a strike, provide proof that the joints can withstand impact and demonstrate psychological commitment to the blow.

5. Shaolin Monk 'Pillar of Skill'

Shaolin monks are known around the world for their incredible feats of mental and physical strength that almost defy the laws of physics and biology. How do they do it? Well, one method is to balance on a pillar (or two pillars) with a large spear pointed at their backside. Should the monk lose balance or focus, he would get a sharp spike in gentlemanly parts to encourage him to re-adopt the proper technique. Developing balance, strength, endurance and pain tolerance at the same time, this may seem brutal but could be considered a mere warm-up compared to the final method of training that also comes from the Shaolin monastery.

6. Shaolin Monk 'Iron Egg'

Shaolin monks are said to possess the strength of an ox, cat-like reflexes and a resolve made of pure steel, making them feared adversaries in any fight. But even the most skilled martial artists can be rendered helpless with a swift kick to the genitals. Yes, it sounds odd I know, but if ever there was a chink in the armour of even the most lethal male fighter, it would be an unprotected pair of testicles. Which is exactly why Shaolin monks practise developing an 'iron egg' by repeatedly taking kicks to the groin in an attempt to toughen up this vulnerable region. Once a monk is able to tolerate a short, sharp kick, they can graduate to a more advanced testicle training technique where sticks, bricks and other objects are used to develop an 'iron crotch'.

Back in the gym, I looked at Dan nervously.

'We're not going to train the "iron egg" today, are we?' I asked.

149

'No,' he replied with a laugh.

He then told me that mixed martial arts training has evolved so much in recent years and that today the periodisation of training draws upon all the insights and analytics from tactical, medical, physical and nutritional domains. The UFC Performance Institute in Nevada, USA even released the first-ever comprehensive study of the sport of MMA in the form of an 80-page report entitled 'A Cross-Sectional Performance Analysis and Projection of the UFC Athlete'. The study involved work with hundreds of UFC athletes that resulted in the collection of over 30,000 performance metrics and data points. From this research, fighters have been able to periodise their training in a manner that represents a dramatic evolution since the days of Pankration in ancient Greece.

THE PERIODISATION OF PANKRATION

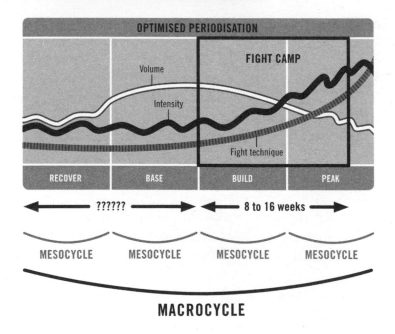

Obviously, every fighter's training camp will be different. A periodised plan must take into account the athlete's level of fitness, injuries, opponent and even how much weight they may need to cut. But (typically) fight camps can be around 8 to 16 weeks and would form part of the *Build* and *Peak Mesocycle*, while the *Recovery* and *Base Mesocycle* can be as long as they want (or need) depending on how many fights per year they have scheduled.

Therefore, represented in a graph (and looking very similar to the periodisation model already used within this book) the only thing that changes is the duration of each mesocycle and the time they take place throughout the year.

Coincidentally, when I arrived at the gym that day I was transitioning from my *Base Mesocycle* to my *Build Mesocycle*. Therefore, in many ways, I was entering into 'fight camp' as we increased the intensity of my training and reduced the volume. This is a very important phase in any periodised plan, because whether you're a swimmer, cyclist, adventurer or fighter it represents a transition where you switch from:

- **General Physical Preparedness to (Sports)** *Specific* **Physical Preparedness**. As you begin to specialise in your chosen sport or activity of your athletic adventure.
- **Work Capacity & Functional Strength to Explosive Strength & Speed.** As you turn the functional strength developed into explosive strength, speed and power.
- **Aerobic Fitness ('gas tank') to Anaerobic Fitness.** As you learn to operate at higher and faster intensities and build on the large 'engine' already built during the *Base Mesocycle* by adding some 'jet engine afterburners'.

Represented in a graph, this *important* transition (from *Base Mesocycle* to *Build Mesocycle*) in your periodised plan looks like this:

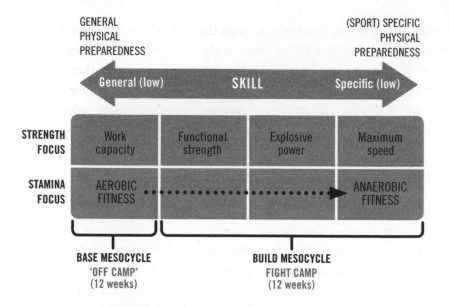

Worth noting is this applies to almost all sports.

Taking inspiration from the world of modern martial arts, I always like to think of this transition phase (from *Base* to *Build Mesocycle*) as getting 'battle ready' as you enter your own 'fight camp' (or Agoge) specific to your sport. You have to essentially lock yourself away, be prepared to sacrifice parts of your social life, become tunnel visioned on your goal and commit to embarking on your athletic adventure.

It sounds cheesy, but this is always my favourite part of every *Rocky* movie!

This is when Rocky Balboa downs a glass of raw eggs in the morning, starts running miles through the streets of Philadelphia, punches dead cows in the meat locker freezer at his local butchers and (most importantly) checks into Mighty Mick's Gym to train under the tutelage of Mickey Goldmill who hurls both instructions and profanities at him.

During my preparation for the Great British Swim in early 2018, I didn't mind checking into Manley Mere after hours and sometimes swimming sprint intervals through the night away from any distractions. With the 'Eye of the Tiger' song often playing on repeat in my head, for me there was a certain romantic ideal about this form of training since everyone's 'fight camp' (regardless of their chosen sport or adventure) should be wrapped in eudaimonia, askēsis and eustress.

Back in the gym I lay on the mat bruised, battered but happy.

'You ok?' Dan asked handing me an ice-pack for my newly swollen lip.

Pressing it against my face to reduce the swelling, but unable to stop smiling, I replied, 'Honestly, I'm so happy. It just feels so good to be back training and hurting again.'

Dan nodded, he knew exactly what I meant. This true 'savage scholar' finds his version of eudaimonia, askēsis and eustress through studying the art of violence and gets so passionate when talking about the discipline, the grind and that feeling of going to war.

For me? I had loved my first maiden voyage into mixed martial arts, but knew that I found true happiness with fulfilment at sea when swimming and suffering in an Arctic storm. So just months after finishing my *Recovery Mesocycle* (to fix my squishy sea feet) and *Base Mesocycle* (to wash off 'spiritual decay' and build a 'gas tank') I was ready to return to the water and check into my own 'fight camp' again. But little did I know this initial return would not be as an athlete or adventurer, but as a coach.

GENERAL PHYSICAL PREPAREDNESS TO (SPORTS) SPECIFIC PHYSICAL PREPAREDNESS

It was mid-spring when I got the email completely out of the blue. It was a media company who were working on a Channel 4 project in the UK to raise money for the charity Stand Up to Cancer.

Immediately, I loved the cause (having worked with the Teenage Cancer Trust years before) but upon reading their email I quickly realised their mission was as noble as it was wildly optimistic:

Dear Ross,
Time is not on our side, so we will get straight to the point.

We have just a few months to train a group of 11 celebrities to swim 21 miles (34 km) across the English Channel in a relay to raise money for charity. The issue we have is many of these celebrities can't actually swim right now and need to learn first. We are aware this is a big ask, but having watched your Great British Swim we know you like an ambitious aquatic adventure and that you understand the British waters better than anyone else, which is why we wanted to contact you to ask if you'd consider coaching our team along with 10-km open water world champion Keri-Anne Payne?

The team will be: Linford Christie (1992, Olympic 100 metres champion), Alex Brooker (comedian), Tessa Sanderson (1984, Olympic javelin champion), Greg Rutherford (2016, Olympic long jump champion), Sair Khan (actress), James 'Arg' Argent (television personality), Georgia Kousoulou (television personality), Simon Webbe (singer), Wes Nelson (television personality), Rachel Adedeji (actress) and Diane Louise Jordan (television presenter).

Please do let us know, since we're aware having you at the proverbial helm would increase our chances of success in completing the swim and raising money for a truly great cause.

I won't lie, at the start of the email I liked the idea, but by the end I loved it. Keri-Anne was a good friend of mine and we'd trained together for years before (she even helped me during my preparation to swim 100 km across the Caribbean Sea towing a 100 lb tree). So, as a fellow coach, I trusted her implicitly.

Also, Linford Christie was a childhood hero of mine. I still remember the men's 100 metres at the 1992 Summer Olympics in Barcelona, Spain, where he ran 9.96 seconds to take gold. Years later and he became my hero as a coach too, when he taught me to run at Brunel University alongside some of Britain's best sprinters. Therefore, to now repay the favour and help him learn to swim was something I was excited and honoured to do.

But the main reason I loved this project was because the entire adventure was basically riddled with eudaimonia, askēsis and eustress. You see, the 21 mile (34 km) stretch of water from Dover to Calais is sacred for all open-water swimmers. First crossed on 25 August 1875 by Captain Matthew Webb, at the time sailors claimed this was swimming suicide because the tides were too strong and the water too cold. But Captain Webb, in a woollen wetsuit and on a diet of brandy and beef broth, swam breaststroke (because 'front crawl was ungentlemanly-like' at the time) and battled waves for over 20 hours to make history. Years later, in 1926 the American-born swimmer Gertrude Ederle (known as 'Queen of the Waves') became the first woman to swim the Channel in a time of 14 hours and 34 minutes and ever since many swimmers have followed in the footsteps of these pioneers.

But worth noting is that everyone who stands on the white cliffs of Dover and looks out to sea in anticipation of their forthcoming cross-Channel swim has been training for many years and many miles to fulfil this lifelong ambition.

No-one had ever attempted this after only learning to swim just months before.

To many observers, this was an ill-fated adventure that should never be attempted. But for me, the reason I loved this so much was because regardless of the outcome, the process (and journey) would be incredible. Yes, if we made it across the celebrations would be biblical and the money we could raise for charity would be immense. But even if we didn't succeed, 11 novices (some with a real fear of the water) would have learned to be competent and capable swimmers.

In short, it was a great cause. So, I accepted the role and later that month prepared to meet the 11 celebrities who'd learn to swim and tackle the English Channel, all in the name of charity and adventure.

SWIMMING BAPTISM: SINK OR SWIM

It was midday at Tinside Lido in Plymouth, England. Perhaps the most quintessential example of a British public pool from a bygone era, it was built in 1935 on a headland overlooking the harbour but still possessed this art-deco style and vintage charm that had remained unchanged for decades. In fact, walking onto the poolside it felt like taking a stroll back through time as the cast-iron railings surrounding the fountains were still immaculately polished and preserved and the fortified concrete walls that had protected the

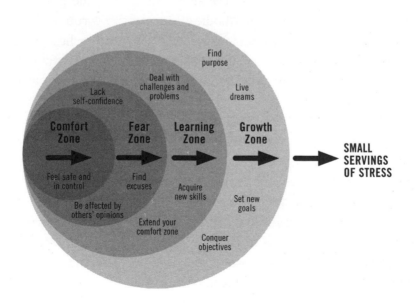

facility from waves, weather and even a world war still looked as impenetrable as the day they were made.

Basically, I loved this form of durable, hardened grandeur. The pool itself was no different either. Created in a semi-circle with a 180 ft (55 m) diameter, it's filled with fresh saltwater directly from the English Channel, which means the temperature is often a lot lower than most swimming pools (28°C/82°F) and today would be around 18°C (65°F). Obviously, this wouldn't be pleasant for my swimming students who were not acclimatised to this, but it was necessary. Almost like a mini-'baptism' to give them just a small serving of eustress to move from their 'comfort zone', past the 'fear zone' and into the 'learning zone'. Of course, some were more willing to get 'baptised' than others, which is why one-by-one myself and Keri-Anne invited them to enter the water so we could assess just how comfortable, competent and capable each member of the team was.

Very quickly, it became apparent everyone had their strengths and weaknesses.

Greg, Linford and Tessa were strong, powerful and genetically blessed and had trained their bodies to jump longer, run faster and throw further at the Olympic Games than any other human. But swimming long distances would require them to completely change their training and mind-set, from fast and powerful to slow and smooth.

Meanwhile Sair, Dianne, Georgia and Rebecca were absolutely fearless and I came to call them my Spartan Sea Sisters. But they had never been taught proper technique, and in sea swimming mental fortitude will only get you so far if it's not coupled with the correct swim stroke.

Next, Wes and Simon both came from a martial arts background, but they'd have to learn to understand that you cannot 'fight' the sea, since you will always lose. Instead, you must learn to glide and dance through the waves and read the tides and currents.

Then we had James 'Arg' Argent who was powerful and very comfortable in the water, but openly (and honestly) admitted he'd never trained for an athletic adventure of this scale, and his life for the last few years had lacked any form of askēsis and eustress.

But none of this mattered, since I truly believe everyone can be taught how to swim. What I wanted to see was a resolute refusal to quit, something embodied by the last swimmer to take to the water, Alex Brooker. Known for his comedy genius, I spoke to him poolside and quickly realised his path to eudaimonia and quest to cross the English Channel was going to be very different and involve a different kind of askēsis. This is because Alex was born with a twisted right leg which had to be amputated when he was a baby. Also, despite spending the first 10 years of his life undergoing hundreds of operations on his hands and upper limbs, he had limited functionality in both hands and a reduced range of motion in his arms.

'You ok, buddy?' I asked.

He nodded, but was clearly worried.

'Hmm . . . yes, it's just swimming lessons at school weren't my favourite,' he said.

'Oh, but you've had lessons?' I asked, happy to hear he had at least some experience.

'Not exactly,' he said.

'During my first swimming lesson at secondary school I was given armbands and made to sit in a canoe without a paddle. As the other kids swam laps of the pool doing various drills, I just spun around at the mercy of the waves that their collective leg kicks created. Ever since, it's just been assumed by most teachers that I'm not very well suited for a sport like swimming.' He said all this while smiling but obviously trying to conceal a memory that was best forgotten.

I paused for a moment.

Angry and upset, I wanted to carefully consider my response to Alex, because the truth is swimming can sometimes be quite narrow-minded and progress over the years has been paralysed by self-imposed rules, regulations and traditions.

But the truth is, there is no correct way to move through the water. In theory it's so simple, you swim by:

- **Achieving Buoyancy.** This is the ability to float in water.
- **Increasing Propulsion.** This is the act of driving, pushing or propelling forward.
- **Reducing Drag.** This is a force that resists and slows forward motion (propulsion).

How Alex achieves this with his body is irrelevant. Basically, there's no right or wrong way and whoever told him he was not 'well suited for a sport like swimming' simply lacked the sporting IQ, imagination and creativity to find a stroke that worked for him and his physiology.

I didn't blame his old swimming teacher either; throughout history swimming has been reluctant to learn and change. In fact, when competitive swimming became popular in England, in 1837 the National Swimming Society (which regulated competition) strongly advocated the use of breaststroke in competition. Any

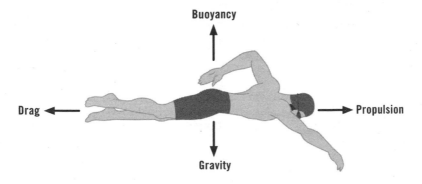

other stroke was considered ungentlemanly and offended Victorian sensibilities at the time. This is despite good evidence that an overarm stroke was used in antiquity by the Assyrians and Greeks and a variety of crawl-style strokes were used by the South Sea Island natives, North American Indians and the Kaffirs of South Africa.

This is why a swim in April 1844 caused such controversy when two Native Americans from the Ojibwe tribe by the names of Flying Gull and Tobacco were invited to the swimming baths in High Holborn, London, to compete in an exhibition race against the Englishman Harold Kenworthy. It's believed the swim was set up to justify an English sense of superiority, so race organisers made the visiting swimmers race each other first. Then (once suitably tired) Kenworthy was able to race and win, 'with the greatest ease' according to the *London Times*.

When commentating on the swimming style of the Ojibwe swimmers, the author wrote, 'Their style of swimming is totally un-European. They lash the water violently with their arms, like the sails of a windmill, and beat downwards with their feet, blowing with force, and fanning grotesque antics.' As a result, British swimmers continued to ignore this style of stroke for another eight years until another pioneer arrived in the form of John Arthur Trudgen who challenged the swimming status quo.

Born in Poplar in 1852, at the age of 11 he went to live in Buenos Aires, Argentina, after his father was relocated for work. During his time there, Trudgen would swim with the local children who used an overarm swimming action rather than the more usual breaststroke. When he returned to England in 1868, he developed the stroke he saw in Argentina and on 11 August 1873, at the Lambeth Baths, London, made swimming history by winning with a style that was unrecognisable to British spectators. Keeping flat on his chest with his head carried high in the air, Trudgen startled onlookers by swinging each arm alternately over the water and making one horizontal breaststroke kick to each cycle of the arms, so that his body lifted and progressed in jerky leaps. One journalist wrote:

> A surprising swimmer carried off the handicap we allude to Trudgen; this individual swam with both arms entirely out of the water, an action peculiar to Indians. His time was very fast, particularly for one who appears to know but little of swimming, and should he become more finished in style, we shall expect to see him take a position almost second to none as a swimmer.
>
> I question, indeed, if the swimming world ever saw a more peculiar stroke sustained throughout a 160 yards race. I have seen many fast exponents retain the action for some distance, but the great exertion compels them to desist, very much fatigued. In Trudgen, however, a totally opposite state of things existed; for here we had a man swimming apparently easy, turning very badly, and when finished, appearing as though he could have gone at least another 80 yards at the same pace. His action reminds an observer of a style peculiar to the Indians, both arms are thrown partly sideways, but very slovenly, and the head kept completely above water.[211]

What Trudgen did at Lambeth Baths was pioneering. Not in terms of the swimming stroke, since (again) there was ample evidence of swimming from ancient civilisations and even artwork found in an Egyptian tomb from around 2000 BCE that shows an overarm stroke like the front crawl. But it was pioneering in the way it encouraged others to think differently and ushered in a new era of scientific stroke analysis to achieve greater speeds over greater distances.

Something the great Cavill family of Australia did better than anyone.

Recognised as the 'first family of Australian swimming',[212] over two generations (in the late nineteenth and early twentieth centuries) their medal tally, collection of trophies and contribution to swimming around the world is hard to quantify. Which is why in 1970, six members of the family were jointly inducted into the International Swimming Hall of Fame. Notably they included Richmond 'Dick' Cavill (the son Richard 'Frederick' Cavill) and Arthur Rowland Channel ('Tums') Cavill who jointly developed the Trudgen stroke to create the Australian crawl and Sydney St Leonards Cavill who was the originator of the butterfly stroke.

Back on poolside with Alex, I wanted to bring back the same innovation, optimism and creativity of Flying Gull, John Trudgen and the Cavill family. Since I truly believe everyone can swim *if* they are encouraged to adopt a style that uniquely works for them, void of rules and preconceived ideas.

Alex sat there in silence, 'digesting' my brief history lesson.

'How do you propose I "increase propulsion" with one leg?' he asked.

I smiled, since he had already begun his own form stroke analysis.

'Glad you asked,' I replied. 'Studies show your leg kick (during front crawl) accounts for 10 to 20 per cent[213] of your overall propulsion and its main role is to keep the body streamlined to reduce drag.[214]

'With a custom-made, tactically fitted prosthetic leg and a stroke we develop entirely specific to you, I honestly believe we can have you gliding through waves from here to France,' I said.

Addressing the group, I then told them that everyone must find a technique that's unique, specific and personal to them. Yes, we must all adhere to the laws of hydrodynamics (the study of objects moving through the water), but today's sports scientists warn about trying to replicate movement images displayed by successful athletes.[215] Research published in the *Scientific Principles for Swimming Techniques* stated that, 'When one considers the differences in lever lengths, the origins and insertions of muscles, the shape of fluid flow about the body, and the actual mind-set that controls the application to swimming techniques, it quickly becomes obvious that no two swimmers should expect to look completely alike when swimming any competitive swimming stroke.'

The *Journal of Swimming Research* wrote, 'It must be recognized that asymmetry is not necessarily associated with a decrease in performance.' Asymmetries are where body parts (and movement) are not equal, in balance or symmetrical. For example, an early study of breaststroke swimmers revealed that technique asymmetry is very common and does not necessarily reduce performance.[216]

So I had each member of the team study the passage below from my book *The Art of Resilience* that explored the sports science of my swim around Great Britain. Detailing the basics of any efficient swimming technique,[217] it is based on the teachings from the *Journal of Swimming Research*[218] and it would become their bible as they learned to develop Specific Physical Preparedness themselves.

*

When considering what variables might affect performance, reference to a model (see figure below) is useful. Resistance and propulsion, together with physiological capacity of the swimmer, are the key determinants of performance.

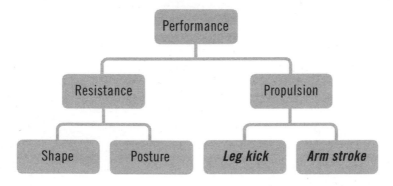

Now 'shape' was obviously different for every member of the team. But something else to consider is posture. It's a fact that most studies on hydrodynamics are limited to objects of regular, symmetrical and unchanging shape. In contrast, the human body is not regular, and constantly changes shape during swimming. What this means is, even an athlete with the perfect 'swimmer's body' will produce irregular shapes that cause drag, whether that's due to the pull and recovery action of the arm or turning to breathe.

Therefore, the overall aim is to maintain a shape that minimises resistance while still positioning the body and its limbs to generate propulsion in an energetically efficient manner. This requires 'trade-offs' to optimise the combination of resistance and propulsion to maximise speed at a sustainable energetic cost. This is why a basic understanding of Newton's laws of motion helps, since they pervade all human movements and cannot be ignored when describing or analysing competitive swimming techniques. Take his first law for example:

Newton's First Law of Motion: A body remains at rest, or continues to move in a straight line at constant velocity, unless acted upon by a net external force.

In swimming, there are forces that accelerate a swimmer, for example the propulsive forces generated by the power-phase in arm strokes, and forces that negatively accelerate a swimmer, for example, resistances and counter-productive movements.

What is a desirable conclusion from this interpretation of Newton's First Law is that propulsive forces should be magnified and applied continuously and that resistive forces should be minimised. That would result in a high level of 'propelling efficiency', and we do this by refining our technique.

EVOLUTION OF THE GREAT BRITISH SWIM

Now, for me, this is where things got interesting. Since when I swam around Britain (2018) I did it with two healthy, fully functioning shoulders where the acromioclavicular (AC) joints were young, healthy and more than happy to rotate millions of times in a single summer. But fast forward 2 years and (although it's hard for me to admit) ever since my surgery I've become painfully aware I'm not a swimming 'spring chicken' anymore, which is why I must substitute youth, strength and stamina for age, wisdom and philosophy.

This approach to swimming was (again) inspired by the martial arts legend Bruce Lee and his creation of Jeet Kune Do. This was a hybrid philosophy for martial arts that was described, 'As a concept, not a style'. This is because he felt that styles such as boxing, Taekwondo and Kung Fu were too formulaic, strict and rigid in their rules and methodology. Instead Lee wanted to teach students to be free from styles, patterns or moulds. He advocated the liberation from styles and patterns believing that real combat is alive and dynamic and real fights don't follow rules and regulations.

This is why through a process of interdisciplinary research, experimentation and innovation, Lee created the 'four ranges of combat' or the four fighting distances (kicking, punching, trapping and grappling). Within these he then developed principles – again, not rules – which he hoped would help guide his students to fight whilst remaining immune to the limitations imposed from martial arts styles.

- The dominant and stronger hand should be the leading hand. Place your stronger side up front. Because the leading hand will perform a greater percentage of the work.
- The best defence is a strong offence.

- Combine defence and attack into one action.
- Avoid telegraphing your punches. Your attack should be unexpected, surprising your opponent.

Ultimately, he wanted his students to be fluid like water, which is why he famously said: 'Empty your mind. Be formless, shapeless. Like water. You put water into a bottle and it becomes the bottle. You put it in a teapot, it becomes the teapot. Water can flow, or it can crash. Be water, my friend!'

In many ways swimming is governed by the same strict styles that governed martial arts in 1967, since coaches (around the world) advocate different styles. From straight-line swimming to the total immersion method, there are hundreds of ways strictly prescribed to move through the water. Which is why (as a coach and swimmer myself) I didn't want to add yet another style to this already exhaustive list. Instead, based on research from the Journal of Swimming Research, I wanted to create the sea swimming version of Jeet Kune Do and create a 'Concept' – not another style – which would allow my students (notably Alex) to create their own unique stroke.

THE AQUATIC ART OF 5 LIMBS

Freestyle (front crawl) remains one of fastest and most efficient ways to achieve buoyancy, increase propulsion and reduce drag in the water. Although the stroke has been refined a lot over the years thanks to pioneers like Flying Gull (from the Ojibwe tribe), John Trudgen and the Cavill family, the basics have remained the same and relatively unchanged and unchallenged.

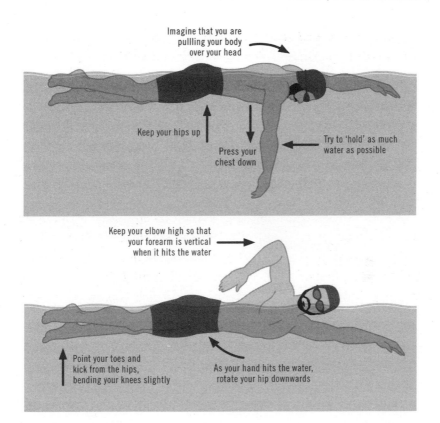

Imagine that you are pullling your body over your head

Keep your hips up

Press your chest down

Try to 'hold' as much water as possible

Keep your elbow high so that your forearm is vertical when it hits the water

Point your toes and kick from the hips, bending your knees slightly

As your hand hits the water, rotate your hip downwards

Body Position	Breathing
Aim to keep your body position as flat as you can to be streamlined in the water with a slight slope down to the hips to keep the leg kick underwater.	Try to keep your head turn as smooth as possible when you breathe. Your neck should remain smooth with your head and spine joining the rotation of the shoulders.
Try to keep your stomach flat and level to support your lower back.	One side of the face should remain in the water and you may want to stretch your mouth to one side to keep it clear.

(continued)

(continued)

Body Position	Breathing
With eyes looking forward and down, your head should be in line with the body and the water level should come between your eyebrows and hairline.	Try not to lift your head too much out of the water – the more your head raises, the more your feet and legs will sink in the water.
Try to keep your head and spine as still and relaxed as possible. Instead, rotate your hips and shoulders to generate momentum through the water. Your head should only join the rotation when you want to breathe.	After a sharp inhale, turn your face quickly and smoothly back into the water in time with the rotation of your shoulders.
Your shoulder should come out of the water as your arm exits while the other begins the propulsive phase under the water.	Exhalation takes place in the water when the head is back to a neutral position and can be gradual or explosive.
The hips should not rotate as much as the shoulders.	The regularity of breathing is not set in stone – it is better to simply inhale when necessary. A standard technique is to breathe every three strokes, thus alternating the side which the head turns and maintaining balance through the stroke.

Arm Stroke	Leg Kick
Keep your elbow slightly bent as you reach your hand in front of your body to enter the water.	Studies show your leg kick (during front crawl) only accounts for 10 to 20 per cent[219] of your overall propulsion and its main role is actually to keep the body in a streamlined position and thereby reduce drag.[220]

(continued)

Arm Stroke	Leg Kick
Entry should be between the centre line of the head and the shoulder line and the hand should be directed with the palm facing down and out so the thumb first enters the water first.	Your legs should be close together with ankles relaxed and in a continuous motion.
Don't start pulling back as soon as your hand is in the water – you should give yourself room to reach forward under the water before you start to bring your hand back to the body.	There's no need to take large down and upbeats – a steady, small motion is fine. While the most pressure should be on your feet, remember to move your whole legs.
The power-phase comes from the pull just above the head and to the hip.	Try to keep your legs as straight as possible. There should be a slight knee bend between the end of the upbeat and beginning of the downbeat but generally the straighter your legs, the more efficient and powerful the kick. The more kicks per cycle, the more energy you will use. Sprint swimmers will typically use six or eight kicks for a cycle, but someone swimming longer distance should use fewer, more pronounced kicks.

But in 2020 I was forced to evolve as an athlete and coach.

This is because my shoulders were still transitioning from the surgery table to the sea which meant I was no longer able to 'muscle my way' through the waves with strength, stamina and sheer stubbornness like I used to. Instead I was forced to find anything and everything I could use to increase propulsion and reduce drag. Not just as a swimmer myself, but as a coach too. This is because I needed to find new ways for Alex to increase propulsion with limited functionality and range of motion in both hands and legs.

This is why I (again) took inspiration from the world of martial arts and began studying Muay Thai. Also known as the 'art of eight limbs' – since it's characterized by the combined use of fists, elbows, knees and shins – it uses any and every limb on the human body as a weapon. Which got me thinking: when swimming many coaches place great emphasis on the arms and legs, but could any other body part be used to aid propulsion? Was I missing a vital component? Sports science says, yes! The fifth (and often forgotten) 'limb' that greatly enhances swimming speed is your core. Effectively engaging (and training) this would help both me and Alex, which is why I coined the term, 'The Aquatic Art of 5 Limbs'.

To understand why, you must understand how the core functions along with research from the National Conditioning Association which stresses a swimmer's core assists power development and propulsion through the hips.[221] It does this since, 'Most movements originate and are transferred through the core to the outer extremities, making it the anchor or reference point of all movement. Unlike ground-based sports in which the ground becomes the reference point of movement, in swimming and other sports that do not require ground contact to direct force the core becomes the point of reference of all movement.'

Sports scientists add: 'In swimming, the arms and the hips are responsible for propelling the body through the water and both are directly connected to the lumbar spine. A strong core will enable more energy to be transferred from the core to the pull and kick components of the stroke. A weak core will allow more energy to leak out, resulting in a less powerful pull and kick.'

Basically, engaging and strengthening the core allows you to transfer energy and develop a more powerful stroke by creating rotation between the hips and shoulders. This is due to the diagonal nature of the muscles in the core working together as a unit in what's known as the Serape Effect.[222]

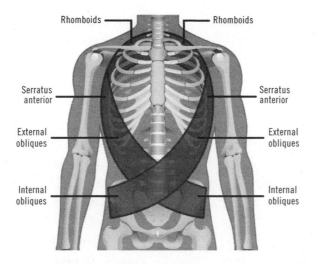

An idea first presented by kinesiologists Gene Logan and Wayne McKinney in 1970, the Serape Effect describes how the internal and external oblique muscles, the rhomboids and the serratus anterior, wrap around the body in an X-pattern (similar to the Mexican serape blanket that is worn around the back of the neck, crosses in the front of the body and tucks into the beltline, hence its name). This diagonal pattern allows the hips to lead and the shoulders to follow in many land-based sports such as throwing, batting or punching[223] and mastery of this kinetic chain power transfer is the reason most elite NFL quarterbacks can throw the ball 70 to 80 yards.

It's also the reason why the boxer with the strongest arm isn't always the boxer with the greatest knockout power. Instead, it's the person who can create power and torque as they 'wind up' the body, unleashing power via the rotary action of the hip via the trunk and the arm. The same is true of the kicking motion too. Because of the criss-cross or 'serape' orientation of the core musculature, the body is able to produce force by connecting the right shoulder to the left hip, and vice-versa.

Exactly the same laws of biomechanics apply to swimming too, as the best swimmers are able to use their core to produce powerful rotational movements very efficiently (during both freestyle and backstroke) as they incorporate something called a 'body roll'. Important to note is that to this day experts still debate how much a swimmer should rotate. Way back in the 1960's there was a trend among the coaching community to teach swimmers to remain as flat as possible (almost like a surfboard). Then during the 1990's this changed and it was encouraged to rotate 90° degrees on the side of every stroke (to 'swim like a fish'). Today many experts state 30° degrees is optimal.

However, I'm reluctant to give such a 'solid' prescription. Doing this would mean I'm creating another style that's too formulaic, strict and rigid in its methodology. Instead – inspired by Bruce Lee and Jeet Kune Do – I was keen to create, 'A concept, not a style' and teach swimmers to be free from styles, patterns or moulds. This is why when I'm asked, 'How many degrees should I rotate?' My answer is, 'However much you individually need to fully utilise the serape effect ... on each arm'. This final point is also so important since for me, I would rotate 30° degrees on my right shoulder but 45° degrees on my left shoulder to help alleviate the pressure on my recovering AC (acromioclavicular) joint. For Alex – when initially training in freestyle – he would rotate 25° degrees to his left and 35° degrees to his right (as he began to use his powerful lats and custom-built prosthetic leg). Were either of us poetic to watch in the water? Probably not. But (again) to quote the *Journal of Swimming Research*, 'It must be recognized that asymmetry is not necessarily associated with a decrease in performance'.

Which is why with all my students I try to empower them to 'feel the water' to know when they're fully utilising the serape effect. To describe it to you now, imagine your hand entering the water. As the right hand enters, your body is rotated/rolled to the left. Then, as you begin the catch (pull phase of the stroke), the body begins the counter-rotation back to the right. This point where the counter-rotation starts is often called the 'connection' between the arm and core (and hips). This counter-rotation creates a stabilizing force for your body and gives you something to pull against so you can exert more force on the water and puts the entire body in a more favourable position to the larger, more powerful muscle groups like the latissimus dorsi muscle (commonly called 'lats') rather than relying solely on the smaller, weaker muscles like the deltoids (shoulders).

Watching this this 'click' as a proverbial lightbulb went off in Alex's was one of the best moments of my coaching career. Since to quote Socrates, 'I cannot teach anybody anything. I can only make them think'. This same advice also applies to everything else in swimming too. From hand placement and kick-to-arm cycle to whether you should breathe bilaterally (both sides) vs unilaterally (only to one side), it's entirely different for everyone and this individual-variability will change even more at sea in a tailwind, headwind or if an angry seal is chasing you.

SWIM LIKE A SPARTAN LEADER

The sun was setting on Plymouth which signalled the end of our first session. As a coach, I couldn't have been more proud. Every member of the team had learned how to achieve buoyancy, increase propulsion and reduce drag. Granted, it wasn't fast and nor was it far, but at least it was a start. This, coupled with their joint refusal to quit meant myself and Keri-Anne had all the 'raw materials' we needed to create a Channel swimming relay team.

I then stressed everyone had homework to do and when they weren't physically swimming, they should be studying it. Analysing stroke technique, they must become scholars of swimming devoted to developing (Sports) Specific Physical Preparedness.

Leading by example, I assured them I would be doing the same. So, once the team headed to the changing room and the media crew packed away their camera equipment, I jumped into the pool and proceeded to swim 10 km.

Taking inspiration (again) from Spartan culture, this was so important. For ancient Spartans, character, honour and virtue were paramount. They didn't trust philosophers or intellectuals, believing that wisdom should be displayed through your actions and the way you live your life. This is why the Spartan king Agasicles once turned away a very learned teacher saying, 'I want to be a pupil of those whose son I should like to be as well.'

This adopted philosophy also explains the life of King Leonidas. Although historians don't have a lot of information about this warrior king of Sparta, we know he was born sometime around 530 to 540 BCE and was tasked with leading a relatively small Greek force to hold the line against a much larger Persian force led by Xerxes at Thermopylae in 480 BCE. The king of Persia had already conquered northern Greece and was on his way to capture the south, but Leonidas bravely defended his position even though his army of just 4,000 soldiers was no match for the 80,000-strong Persian force.

They fought to the death, a statue of Leonidas stands in his homeland of Sparta to honour his great courage and his story has since been immortalised in the modern film *300* (released in 2006). The most iconic line was when a Spartan soldier turns to Leonidas and says, 'It's an honour to die at your side' to which the warrior king replies, 'It's an honour to have lived at yours.'

Inspired by the man, the king and the legend, I then led the team to the north of England in search of colder lakes, eustress and swimming askēsis and promised that as harsh as the conditions would become, I would never ask them to do anything I wouldn't do myself.

AEROBIC FITNESS ('GAS TANK') TO ANAEROBIC FITNESS

It was somewhere between spring and summer at Lake Windermere. England's largest lake and located in Cumbria's Lake District National Park, it is 10.5 miles long (almost 17 km) and at its deepest point is 219 feet (66.7 m). In many ways, this is sacred water for English Channel swimmers who arrive from all over the world to train since the 16°C (61°F) water temperature closely resembles the conditions found between Dover and Calais.

Basically, this was the ideal setting for the team's first open-water swim.

The team had graduated from the Lido in Plymouth after leaving their 'comfort zone'. But now, with the summer fast approaching and therefore our 'weather window' to cross the Channel getting shorter, I needed them to swim further and learn faster. This meant we needed to leave the 'fear zone' entirely and start living within the 'learning zone' and 'growth zone'.

To do this we would be travelling up and down the country in search of lakes, lochs and open sea as we left the comfort of swimming pools behind. But when doing this with a group of athletes who had only just learned to swim, safety was paramount.

So, before we began I stood on the pontoon overlooking Lake Windermere and took the team through safety signals and spoke about the risks of hypothermia, cold water shock and a loss of feeling and function in the hands and feet. As I did I could sense the nervous energy was practically palpable, but thankfully our team had a secret weapon and it came in the form of Alex Brooker who had a unique way of making everyone smile, irrespective of the situation.

'Ross?' I heard a voice from the back of the group (it was Alex).

'Yes, what's up, brother?' I asked.

'What about me?'

'What about you?' I replied confused.

'Do I need to be worried about a loss of feeling and function in my feet?' he said, pointing to his plastic prosthetic leg.

Everyone burst out laughing and despite completely ruining my safety briefing, I didn't mind. In fact, I encouraged it since Alex possessed a trait that could prove invaluable to the team. It's something the Royal Marines call 'cheerfulness in the face of adversity' and it's formed part of their motto for years because they realise there's great power in smiling even under the most adverse conditions.

This was an idea supported by a study published in the *Journal Psychology of Sport and Exercise* too.[224] Researchers had 24 runners (men and women) complete four 6-minute intervals at 70 per cent maximal effort with 2-minute intervals of rest in between as their oxygen consumption was measured. During each run, volunteers were asked to either smile, scowl, relax or simply fall back on their usual endurance mind-sets while researchers also asked them to rate how they felt and report their coping strategies (for example, whether were they ignoring their pain or embracing it). After analysing the results, it was found that:

- Smiling improved running economy (technique) by 3 per cent compared to frowning.
- Runners consumed less oxygen and are better able to remain aerobic.
- Perceived effort was higher when frowning in comparison with smiling and relaxing.

This last point was particularly relevant. That's because today's training session was not going to be pleasant and with safety briefings done and tension suitably broken (thanks to Alex) I told the team we needed to increase their anaerobic fitness by swimming a series of uncomfortably fast sprints, with very brief periods of rest, between the pontoon and the floating buoys that were 100 m apart as I kept a close eye on the intervals, speed and rest period from the boat.

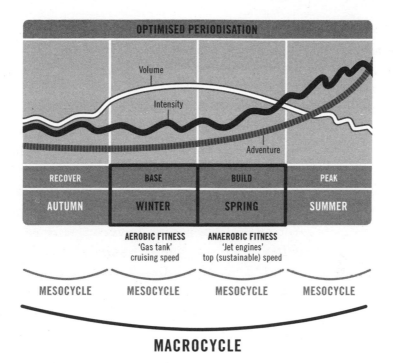

MACROCYCLE

Within a periodised macrocycle, this is the point where the intensity of training increases, but the volume of training slightly decreases since (in theory) a solid aerobic base ('gas tank') has been built during the *Base Mesocycle*. Therefore, your heart, lungs, cardiorespiratory and body as a whole is good when training at low intensity for long periods of time (remember Zone 2 training at 60 to 70 per cent of your maximum heart rate). But now during the *Build Mesocycle* the goal should be to condition the body to work more efficiently at high intensities (adding 'jet engine afterburners' where you operate above your anaerobic threshold and train in Zone 4 (80 to 90 per cent of your maximum heart rate) and if possible Zone 5 (90 to 100 per cent of your maximum heart rate).

This holistic approach to training the body's cardiorespiratory system through the year is based on research from the *International Journal of Sports Physiology and Performance*[225] which found

177

'high-intensity resistance training in the *competitive* phase is likely to produce beneficial gains in performance'. The reason they stated 'competitive phase' is because they understood how each mesocycle must work in synergy to (jointly) improve your body's ability to use both the aerobic energy system (at low intensity) and anaerobic energy system (at high intensity) to provide enough energy to continue to operate whatever the pace of the hike, run or cycle. This is why high-intensity interval training is mainly introduced in the *Build Mesocycle*, and only after a successful *Base Mesocycle* has been completed.

Note this is a method of training that's only been perfected since the 1900s. Prior to that, it was thought to become a good endurance runner you simply had to run many slow, long and hard miles. But in 1910, famed Finnish runner Paavo Nurmi pioneered interval training and used it to set 22 official world records at distances between 1,500 metres and 20 kilometres, win 9 gold and 3 silver medals in his 12 events in the Olympic Games and basically dominate distance running in the early twentieth century. In fact, at his peak the 'Flying Finn' was undefeated for 121 races at distances from 800 metres upwards and throughout his 14-year career remained unbeaten in cross-country events and the 10,000 metres.

Many sports historians credit Nurmi's incredible achievements to his meticulous and almost mathematical approach to running. Famously, he rarely ran without a stopwatch in his hand. The sports commentator Archie Macpherson stated that, 'With the stopwatch always in his hand, he elevated athletics to a new plane of intelligent application of effort and was the harbinger of the modern scientifically prepared athlete.'

But Nurmi didn't just plan his individual training sessions (microcycles) with military precision. No, he had his entire season (macrocycle) mapped out too. In his book *The Kings of Distance: A Study of Five Great Runners*, author Peter Lovesey says that Nurmi 'Accelerated the progress of world records; developed and actually came to personify the analytic approach to running; and he was a profound influence not only in Finland, but throughout the world of athletics. Nurmi, his style, technique and tactics were held to be infallible, and really seemed so, as successive imitators in Finland steadily improved the records.'

For sea swimmers (and most adventurers) this is also so important, since the intensity and pace of the swim is often not dictated by you, but by Mother Nature and Poseidon. What I mean by this is you might be happy swimming at 2 knots (2.3 mph) but if the tide changes against you and is running at 2 knots in the opposite direction, you better hope that you've trained your aerobic and anaerobic energy system enough to operate at different intensities. I warned the team that this can happen during sea swims and if it does they would have three choices:

- You swim at 2 knots, match the speed of the tide and therefore hold your position hoping the tide eventually changes and you can continue to make progress.
- You swim faster than 2 knots and are capable of 'powering through' the current and will make progress against the tide.
- You swim slower than 2 knots and you, together with the rest of us, are pushed back to Dover.

I then warned everyone that this isn't uncommon in the English Channel either. Especially when arriving at Cap Gris Nez in France (the headland halfway between Calais and Boulogne) where the tides are so unpredictable. In fact, there are many reports of swimmers less than a mile away from France who, after over 20 miles of swimming, are pushed back towards Dover by the changing current. Those who had a strong anaerobic fitness capacity were able to break through the tide and finish, but many who were unable to swim at a higher intensity couldn't and were pulled from the water and their attempt was deemed over as they were essentially swimming backwards.

I then stressed to the team that the tides *would* impact on our swim.

It's an unavoidable truth, but how much it impacted on us would depend on the strength of our swimming. The reason being that the shortest distance in a straight line from England to France is 21 miles, but during this crossing the tide changes every six hours, taking the swimmer 'up' the Channel for six hours and 'down' the Channel for six hours. This up and down movement of the water is relentless and unavoidable and could add hours and miles onto our attempt as the tides would force us to tackle a sort of S-shaped course.

Silence (again) from the team.

The magnitude of the task at hand was now painfully evident and the tension previously broken was now back. Standing at the back of the group was Linford deep in thought. One of the world's greatest athlete-turned-coach hybrids within the realm of athletics, his sporting IQ was incredible and you could see he was doing the maths in his head.

'So how far will we swim?' Linford asked.

I paused to consider my response, since the fundamental difference between being an athlete and an adventurer is that the conditions are wildly different as you operate outside of the realms, rules and regulations of conventional sport.

'The truth is, I don't know,' I replied. 'Mother Nature will decide on the day and she might even change it mid-swim. The best way I can describe it to you is like this: imagine you sign up to run a marathon, but then halfway through your quest to run 26.2 miles you find out the race organisers have moved the finish line and turned it into a 50-mile ultra-marathon.'

To illustrate my point, I then showed the team the routes of three different successful swims across the English Channel each of which had to tackle an S-shaped course due to the tides (notice how all were successful, but some had to swim further and for longer than others).

But speed isn't just needed for success, it's need for survival.

This might sound dramatic, but adding hours onto the swim wouldn't just decrease our chances of success, it could also increase the chances of death. Although the exact number of fatalities isn't known, the Channel Swimming & Piloting Federation lists eight deaths between 1926 and 2013 and the Channel Swimming Association lists seven (including three who weren't swimming under the organisation's supervision or seeking its certification).

The exact causes of death are unknown, but one rare and fatal phenomenon that's been reported in sea swimming (that's not shared by other sports) is the ability of some swimmers to compete when in a semi-conscious state. This is because according to research published in the *British Journal of Sports Medicine*[226] once the core body temperature reaches 91°F (32.7°C) and below, respiration and heart rate begin to slow to dangerous levels and we can

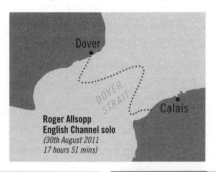

Roger Allsopp
English Channel solo
(30th August 2011
17 hours 51 mins)

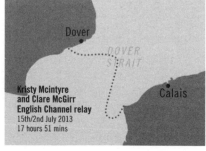

Kristy Mcintyre
and Clare McGirr
English Channel relay
15th/2nd July 2013
17 hours 51 mins

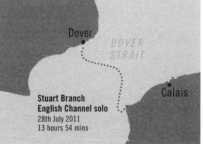

Stuart Branch
English Channel solo
28th July 2011
13 hours 54 mins

lose consciousness. But it's been shown that the muscles can function in temperatures as low as 81°F (27.2°C). That means someone who is very well acclimatised to cold water, has incredible willpower and also has swimming technique and biomechanics 'burned' into their muscle memory, can in theory swim (for a period) beyond the point at which their brain is functioning and they are fully conscious.

It's believed one famous swimmer who did just that was Jason Zirganos. A major in the Greek army and decorated by King Paul in 1949 for being the first Greek ever to swim the English Channel, he was one of the great open-water swimmers of the mid-twentieth century whose tolerance for the cold was legendary and studied by scientists.[227] But one thing that baffled experts was his inability to perceive the dangerous dropping of his own core body temperature.

In 1953, he swam in the Bosphorus (8°C) for four hours. He was removed from the water semi-conscious, regaining full consciousness three hours later. As he was unaware of hypothermia and did not feel particularly cold, it was assumed that he had been poisoned. A year later, at the age of 46, Zirganos attempted to swim the 22-mile North Channel of the Irish Sea (9.4°C–11.7°C). After six hours, and only three miles from the Scottish coast, Zirganos became unconscious and blue; he did not feel 'cold' prior to this. He was hauled from the water and a doctor, using a penknife, exposed Zirganos's heart to reveal ventricular fibrillation. Direct heart massage having failed, Jason Zirganos was pronounced dead at the scene.

'This is why today's session will be painful,' I said.

Members of the team could be seen to visibly wince.

'Not because I want it to be, but because based on everything I have mentioned we *need* it to be,' I added, assuring them it was for their own good.

I then explained about the *Five-Zone Model of Endurance Training* (as explained in the **Build a Bigger Engine** section of the *Base Mesocycle* chapter) and how today's session would be a scaled-down version of the workout I complete three to five times per week during my *Build Mesocycle*.

	Intervals	Rest	Intensity
Warm-Up	500 metres	Irrelevant	Zone 2 *60–70 per cent of your maximum heart rate*
Technique	5 x 200-metre intervals	90 seconds	Zone 3 *70–80 per cent of your maximum heart rate*
Main Set	10 x 200-metre intervals	30 seconds	Zones 4 and 5 *80–100 per cent of your maximum heart rate*
Cool-Down	500 metres	Irrelevant	Zones 1 and 2 *50–60 per cent of your maximum heart rate*

TAKING THE PLUNGE

Standing on the boat on Lake Windemere, I watched as the team members entered the water. As instructed, they each took a moment to acclimatise and control their 'cold shock' response. Then once (and only once) breathing was under control, I told them to begin a slow and steady 500-metre swim (in Zone 2) around the giant, yellow floating buoys while paying attention to their new surroundings.

This last part was particularly important. In fact, it was just as important as the warm-up itself. That's because this was their first time outside the safety of a pool and swimming in an open-water lake, which meant wind, waves and wildlife were all new variables to consider as they focused on achieving buoyancy, increasing propulsion and reducing drag.

Of course, some adapted to their new surroundings better than others.

With no lanes or pool markings to 'sight-off' I had to quickly 'shepherd' Tessa and Diane away from oncoming boats as they swam blindly (and directly) into their path. Meanwhile, a few floating buoys away, Greg was learning to turn his head to breathe and sight-off the trees on the horizon but had managed to ingest most of the lake in the process. All the time, Alex was trying to decide if it was a reed, eel or fish that was stroking his left bum cheek.

Thankfully, after a nail-biting few minutes, the warm-up was complete. So, I instructed the team to return to the pontoon where we'd have a debrief on their maiden voyage into open-water swimming and try to determine what was actually caressing Alex's buttocks.

'So, how did it feel?' I asked, eager to hear what they thought.

'Ok,' was the joint response with a collective shrug of the shoulders before they voiced their concern that the tide had been pulling them 'off course'.

I stood there silent for a moment. I wanted to be sure my response didn't discourage them further since lakes don't have tides or currents, so whatever was 'pulling' the team in the wrong direction was a mystery to me (and sailing science). Therefore, deciding it was best to ignore the fictitious, unidentified rip tide of Lake Windermere for now, I assured them they were doing great. Yes, it wasn't pretty and Greg was still burping from the litres of lake water he'd drunk, but there were definite signs of swimming (buoyancy plus propulsion).

So, after a 'pep talk' I convinced them to get back in the water.

This time they would be performing 5 x 200-metre 'technique' intervals at just above the anaerobic threshold (the point when your body must switch from your aerobic energy system to your anaerobic energy system). The goal here was to train in Zone 3 (70 to 80 per cent of your maximum heart rate) but with lots of rest (90 seconds) between each interval, since it's at this pace where swimming technique can be practised efficiently (Specific Physical Preparedness) working on a streamlined body position, powerful pull with the hands and smooth rotation with the hips and shoulders.

Immediately, you could see a noticeable difference.

Now operating with greater speed, intensity and propulsion the team were no longer being bullied by the imaginary currents and were even able to plough through the giant bow waves created from large passing boats. Smiling and swimming with a restored sense of confidence, I told them they were now ready for their main set, consisting of:

- 10 x 200-metre intervals.
- 30 seconds rest in between.
- Operating in Zones 4 and 5 (80 to 100 per cent of their maximum heart rate).

This would not only bring about physiological changes in anaerobic fitness, but give me a great indication of individual members':

- Top swimming speed.
- Their ability to sustain a faster pace at a higher intensity for longer periods of time.

Inspired by the great Paavo Nurmi, I stood on the boat with my stopwatch in hand ready to monitor their swims and do the maths on their speeds.

Feeling nervous, I knew this session would make or break a lot of them as their bodies were about to be plunged into physiological disarray as:

- Oxygen use increases.
- Heart rates elevate.

- Fuel (muscle glycogen) is burned.
- Chemicals build up in the muscles which contribute to exhaustion.
- Water is lost and heat accumulates.
- Muscles fatigue as the molecular energy of the muscles (adenosine triphosphate) runs low.

As predicted, by the second interval the cracks were beginning to show. In fact, these proverbial cracks were turning into a giant, distinct chasm that separated members of the squad. On the one hand, some members of the team were perfectly happy visiting Zones 4 and 5 and eudaimonia, askēsis and eustress were familiar friends. Take Greg Rutherford, for example, the 2012 Olympic long-jump champion whose powerful legs were the result of over a decade of speed, power and plyometric conditioning. Or Tessa Sanderson the 1984 Olympic javelin champion who in 1996 became the second track and field athlete to compete at six Olympic Games.

Throughout their athletic careers they'd essentially made a holiday home in Zones 4 and 5, so although swimming was a new skill, the ability to systematically endure suffering to improve anaerobic fitness was not.

In contrast, for other members of the squad Zone 4 was a place they'd rarely visit and Zone 5 was an entirely foreign, far-away land they'd never even heard of. Which explains why by the third sprint interval, James Argent was hiding behind a floating buoy hoping that I wouldn't notice.

'Arg!' I shouted.

'You are terrible at hide and seek,' I said.

'Sorry, you got me. It seemed like a good idea,' he replied.

Strangely, I did admire his honesty. He'd openly told me beforehand he'd lived solely within the confines of his comfort zone for years and he hoped this swim, as well as raising money for charity, would serve as a catalyst to help him break out of it. That's why I didn't feel bad for what I did during the third and fourth interval. Peeling his hands away from the pontoon as he clung to the side gasping for air, I wouldn't say I kicked him, but I would say I 'encouraged him to swim with my foot'.

By the fifth (and final) sprint their bodies were riddled with fatigue, but also wrapped in eudaimonia. They all finished sore but smiling, and although they felt like they'd been run over by a tugboat I couldn't have been prouder of each of them.

'Is my anaerobic fitness improved yet?' Alex asked semi-seriously.

'Yes, how many more sessions until we notice a difference?' Arg asked, eager for answers.

Again, I thought about my response carefully. Obviously, any improvement will greatly depend (and vary) on the individual, but I wanted to give them some good news that would prove each painful interval was worth it. So, sitting on the pontoon overlooking the lake and wrapped in towels, I told the team about research published in the journal of *Medicine & Science in Sports & Exercise* that studied the impact of six weeks of high-intensity interval training (eight sets of 20-second intervals with 10 seconds rest in between, performed five times per week) had on aerobic[228] and anaerobic fitness.[229] What they found was, 'Anaerobic capacity increased by 28%' but interestingly they added, 'High-intensity intermittent training may improve *both* anaerobic and aerobic energy supplying systems significantly, probably through imposing intensive stimuli on both systems.'

But interestingly, this wasn't the only physiological adaptation they'd started within their bodies. They had also begun to increase their muscles' 'buffering capacity'.[230] During intense periods of competition or adventure there is a biochemical imbalance within the body which contributes to exhaustion.[231] Studies show that in untrained individuals this can cause the body to fatigue, fail and stop functioning. But in trained athletes and adventurers, the cellular environment within our muscles possesses a buffering-capacity system[232] to help combat this, meaning we can continue to swim oceans, climb mountains and compete at the highest level.[233]

With this 'silver lining' of sports science communicated to the team, they sensed today's training session was worth it and every member of the team left the lake that day with a newfound understanding of askēsis-based interval training in open water swimming having now visited Zones 4 and 5 in England's largest lake.

But after looking at my stopwatch, there was a problem.

That's because today's session was a success in *almost* every sense of the word. Every member of the team had showed courage, grit, determination and a resolute refusal to quit. Also, considering many had only learned to swim weeks before, what they did today was incredible. Unfortunately, today's session lacked one thing . . . *speed*.

Turning to Keri-Anne and the media crew, I could see they knew this too.

Moments later, the team suffered its first casualty in the form of Georgia Kousoulou. Very aware that her top swimming speed wasn't fast enough for the English Channel, she selflessly decided to withdraw herself from the challenge for the good of the team. With her head held high after overcoming a childhood fear of the water, she was the first to leave the team, but (unfortunately) I knew she wouldn't be the last.

TOP-SECRET SWIMMING MISSION

It was 7 p.m. and the sun was beginning to set on Lake Windermere. The team had boarded the bus and headed back to the hotel in search of food, a shower and sleep, and the only people that remained were producers, cameramen and sound technicians from the media crew who were packing up the equipment. Then you had me. Unable to leave until I'd crunched the numbers on our chances of success, I was sitting cross-legged under a tree overlooking the lake writing down the swimming speeds of each member of our team.

Moments later, I was joined by Caroline, executive producer of the entire project.

'How's it looking?' she asked looking concerned.

'Hmm . . . not great,' I replied.

I then showed her the stopwatch and explained how the top speed I recorded today was 1.3 mph (2.1 km/h) and the slowest speed recorded was 0.6 mph (1 km/h). Of course, for a group of novice, inexperienced swimmers this was something to be proud of and should be celebrated, but for anyone wanting to swim the English Channel it was not fast enough and (as a coach) I needed to be honest and realistic. That's because although the crossing is only 21 miles (34 km) across, when swimmers are forced to swim in an S-shape (due to the tides) the final distance covered could be anywhere between 21 miles and 31 miles.

That means with an average speed of 0.95 mph (1.5 km/h), it's possible we could be swimming for more than 30 hours, making us contenders for the slowest crossing of the English Channel. A record currently held by Jackie Cobell, who in 2010 swam a total of 105 km (65 miles) in 28 hours and 44 minutes after being pushed off course by strong tides.

Caroline looked out pensively across the lake. As an experienced open-water swimmer herself, she understood that speed, statistics and the stopwatch were not in our favour, but (like me) refused to admit defeat having become so invested in the project.

'There is one solution,' she said.

'What's that?' I asked, keen to hear any glimmer of hope.

'You were swimming between 2.5 and 3.1 mph (4 and 5 km/h) around Great Britain, right?' she asked.

'Hmm . . . yes, but I've not been seriously training since I arrived back on land,' I confessed (having only really completed a *Recovery* and *Base Mesocycle*).

'So, if you joined the team our average speed would be *a lot more* than 0.95 mph (1.5 km/h) and our chances of arriving in Calais would improve dramatically,' she said.

I stood there in silence, considering the proposed solution.

It certainly made logical sense, since based purely on statistics it would increase our chances of success. But as a coach, and someone studying the science and psychology of *Adventure*, I was worried they would never achieve eudaimonia (through askēsis) if I was to swim a big 'chunk' of their relay for them. Battling with my decision, I then told Caroline I would begin training in secret, but we both agreed that my involvement was a last resort and a contingency plan that we never wanted to use.

By 9 p.m. the lake was entirely empty and the sun had set. Cameras had been loaded into vans, boats had been stored in the boatyard and I was now standing by the lake in my trunks and goggles. Ready to swim into the night, visiting Zones 4 and 5 in my own form of askēsis-based interval training, all in the hope that I would improve anaerobic fitness and develop Specific Physical Preparedness.

All for a swim that I hoped I would never have to do.

WORK CAPACITY & FUNCTIONAL STRENGTH TO EXPLOSIVE STRENGTH & SPEED

It was the morning after my secret swim in Lake Windermere. The team were still unaware that I was covertly training and I was keen for it to stay that way, because if they learned I was joining the relay I feared it would impact on their training, adventure and quest for eudaimonia. This is why I continued to coach through the day but train during the night away from any witnesses and cameras.

As a result, early morning strength sessions and late-night swims became normal, which explains why I was creeping into the hotel gym at 6 a.m. before they woke up, camera crews assembled and we had our team briefing over breakfast.

As a sea swimmer, I understood how the ocean can serve as your judge, jury and executioner. What I mean by this is, if you've missed training sessions, failed to prepare or take a swim too lightly, Poseidon and Mother Nature will find a way to humble you, no matter how strong a swimmer you are.

This is a lesson I learned the hard way in 2017 when I was swimming in the Caribbean Sea, at midnight, with a 100 lb tree attached to my trunks as the crew tried to decide if the shark-dolphin hybrid following me was friend or foe.

Yes, this story is as odd as it sounds.

In November, I had travelled to the Caribbean island of St Lucia with a plan to swim 40 km (24.8 miles) to the neighbouring island of Martinique towing a tree to raise money for environmental charities. It seemed like a good idea at the time, but as the clock struck midnight, and the moon set high in the sky, the tide took a turn for the worse.

'You're being pushed back by the tide,' Vincent (the captain) shouted from the boat.

He'd been sailing these waters for 40 years and knew the volatility and unpredictability of that stretch of water between the two islands where the North Atlantic and Caribbean Sea currents collided.

'You need to swim hard for four hours,' he said, now shining a light from the bow of the boat and pointing in the direction of Martinique.

'Do this and you'll break into more favourable water.'

Taking a deep breath, I knew he was right. Although I'd already swum over 30 km (18.5 miles) I knew no one could help me, so I tightened the tree to my trunks and began swimming as hard as I could. Hours passed and despite my arms being riddled with fatigue and with no concept of how far or fast I was swimming (being engulfed in complete darkness) I continued to battle the waves through the night with blind optimism.

Stroke after stroke, my armpits began to chafe from the saltwater until eventually I could see the sun beginning to rise on the horizon. This was the glimmer of hope I needed since it signalled I had been swimming for close to four hours.

Turning to Vincent, I asked, 'How are we doing? What's our speed? How far left?'

Vincent couldn't look me in the eyes. Standing at the helm of the boat, he reluctantly replied, 'You've not moved.'

'You've been swimming on the same spot for four hours just pushing against the tide.'

Feeling physically exhausted, I was now psychologically wounded too. It was like the ocean was toying with me. If this was a fight, it would be like giving someone your best right uppercut and connecting cleanly to the chin, only to have them laugh it off and continue smiling. As I floated there for a second, I considered my options.

'You could cut the rope, lose the tree and continue without it,' Vincent said.

'I can't,' I replied semi-delirious from fatigue and saltwater.

'What about the orangutans?' I asked.

Vincent looked at me and then the team medic aboard the boat. With worry written across his face, he thought I'd lost my mind at sea and was clearly deciding how best to end the swim and get me and the tree back aboard the boat.

Seeing his concern, I quickly realised I needed to explain myself, so told him I had raised thousands of pounds for charity working to combat deforestation in the Borneo jungle as orangutans were losing their homes. The tree I was towing was symbolic of that. Finishing the swim without it didn't seem right.

'Oh, oh, I see,' he replied with a sigh of relief that I hadn't gone completely mad.

'But right now, we have a bigger problem,' he said.

'What's that?'

'You know the entire time you've been telling me about the orangutans in Borneo?'

'Yes.'

'Well, you've actually been pushed back 300 metres by the tide,' he said.

I then yelled a profusion of profanities that echoed across the Caribbean Sea before putting my face back in the water to do battle with the tides once again. This continued through the day and night, and although I had originally planned to swim 40 km (24.8 miles) I ended up covering over 100 km (62 miles) while dragging the 100 lb tree (which doesn't include the four hours I spent swimming on the spot). Arriving back on land having swum over twice the planned distance, I had a newfound respect for the ocean and vowed that if ever I became involved in another 'fight' with the sea, I would add more tools to my arsenal.

What tools? Well, remember the car engine analogy where:

- My aerobic energy system is like my primary 'gas tank' which I rely on for a slow and steady speed in cruise control mode.
- My anaerobic energy system is like my 'jet engine afterburners' or nitrous oxide engine (NOS) which I use to accelerate.

Well, explosive strength and speed training is like adding more gears to your car.

More gears in a car means you can accelerate faster and you've better fuel economy. Basically, it improves the efficiency of your engine and the same is true of your body and specifically your muscles.

To understand this, you must first understand that sports science teaches us there are two types of muscle fibres. These are **Type I fibres** and **Type II fibres** (Type II fibres can also be further subdivided into Type IIa and Type IIb).

Now, Type I fibres (more commonly known as 'slow twitch' muscle fibres) are great for endurance and essential to get through the Tour de France or London Marathon. These are much more resistance to fatigue. Type II muscle fibres are more commonly known as 'fast twitch' muscle fibres and these are needed to power up the hills during a steep ascent (or in my case, break through tides with a tree attached to your trunks to raise money charity) since they have a faster contractile speed.

How do you build more of these?

In short, through a specific form of speed and strength training. This is why the *Scandinavian Journal of Medicine and Science in Sport* stated, 'Concurrent strength/endurance training in young elite competitive cyclists led to an improved 45-minute time-trial endurance capacity that was accompanied by an increased proportion of type IIA muscle fibre.'[234]

Next, if you move better you move further.

As we discussed before, when it comes to swimming performance the Department of Applied Mechanics and Engineering at Sun Yat-Sen University in China found technique, stroke rate and efficiency will also play a key role[235] (the same is true of other sports too) and it seems strength training is a great tool to help this. According to the *Scandinavian Journal of Medicine and Science in Sport*, 'Adding heavy strength training improved cycling performance (by an) improved cycling economy (movement and efficiency).'[236]

Ultimately, this is why the *European Journal of Applied Physiology* found that, 'Adding strength training to usual endurance training improved determinants of (endurance) performance'[237] since athletes added 'gears' to their 'gas tank' and 'jet engine afterburners.'

Corroborating this theory, the *American Journal of Physiology* stated that, 'These results provide novel insight into human muscle adaptations . . . and offer the very first genomic basis explaining how aerobic exercise may augment (improve), rather than compromise, muscle growth induced by resistance exercise.'[238]

But which form of strength training is best for adding 'gears'?

Well, first you must understand the subtle differences between the different forms of strength and how speed and strength are interlinked. In sports science, strength is defined as your muscles' ability to generate force. Put more simply, this is how much weight you can move during a squat, bench, deadlift or any movement.

But we also understand that strength (your ability to generate force) and speed (your ability to move fast) have an inverse relationship. What this means is, as you put more weight on the bar you increase the force, but you reduce the speed (since you're unable to move the bar as fast). This is what's known as the Force-Velocity Curve and in a graph, it's represented like this:

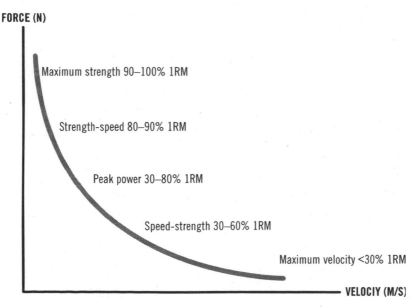

FORCE (N)

Maximum strength 90–100% 1RM

Strength-speed 80–90% 1RM

Peak power 30–80% 1RM

Speed-strength 30–60% 1RM

Maximum velocity <30% 1RM

VELOCIY (M/S)

It is within this graph where the subtle differences in forms of strength are found.

Very similar to the Five-Zone Model of Endurance Training, this is essentially the Five-Zone Model of Strength Training, and whichever zone you choose to visit will depend on the physiological adaptations you want and the physiological adaptations the adventure requires.

MAXIMUM STRENGTH TRAINING ZONE

Training in this zone requires big and heavy weights. Typically, sessions are high intensity, low volume and will include lots of rest between sets to allow you to lift at 90 to 100 per cent of your 1RM performing around 1 to 4 repetitions. The best example of this is a pure, old-school powerlifting programme where athletes squat, bench and deadlift with as much iron on the bar as they can possibly lift.

STRENGTH-SPEED TRAINING ZONE

Training in this zone requires you to lift big and heavy weights, but at speed. This is because strength-speed training requires an athlete to move less weight than is required when training for maximum strength, but move it at a faster speed. The best example of this would be an Olympic lifting session where you're using weight that's 80 to 93 per cent of your 1RM.

PEAK POWER TRAINING ZONE

Training in this zone means you focus equally on speed and strength. Delivering peak power output, these exercises produce the greatest amount of force in the least amount of time and examples include the pull variations of the Clean and Snatch, jump squats and medicine ball throws at 50 to 70 per cent of your 1RM.

SPEED-STRENGTH TRAINING ZONE

Training in this zone requires you to train speed, but with weight. The goal is to move faster than we do during *Strength-Speed Training* with 40 to 60 per cent of your 1RM. Examples include plyometric drills like high hurdle jumps, light-loaded jump squats and battle rope variations, but the focus is on speed rather than strength.

MAXIMAL VELOCITY TRAINING ZONE

Training in this zone requires you to move the body, muscles and joints fast as possible. This type of training can be very sport specific, but let's take sprinting as an example. Running 100 m as fast as you can, will represent 100 per cent of your maximum speed, but perform that same 100 m sprint downhill and therefore assisted (known as 'supramaximal sprinting') and you're now performing above your 100 per cent maximum speed. This training zone is often classified as being at less than 30 per cent of your 1RM.

YOUR STRENGTH AND SPEED TRAINING

So, what part of the Force-Velocity Curve should *you* train in?

Well, that depends on many factors including time, resources, equipment, biological age and many more. But two of the biggest things to consider when designing a strength/speed programme for an adventure are:

- Specific strength and speed qualities of your adventure.
- Your Dynamic Strength Index. This is how we measure the difference between an athlete's maximal strength (like their one repetition maximum squat) and their ballistic strength which is

an athlete's ability to produce force at speed in a short timeframe (like an explosive, weighted vertical jump).

But let's begin by analysing the most obvious: your adventure's strength/speed qualities.

YOUR ADVENTURE'S STRENGTH AND SPEED QUALITIES

Different adventures will require different strength/speed qualities. It seems pretty obvious that you wouldn't programme and prioritise a 180 kg bench press into your strength training routine if, for example, you're training to cycle the 4,400 km (2,734 miles) of the Great Divide Mountain Bike Route from Canada's Alberta all the way to New Mexico in the USA.

No instead, you'd target lower body and core strength.

This is why when analysing the performance of elite cyclists, the *Scandinavian Journal of Medicine and Science in Sport* wrote, 'Adding strength training to usual endurance training improves leg strength and 5-minute all-out performance following 185 minutes of cycling in well-trained cyclists.'[239]

It also added, 'It is concluded that strength training can lead to enhanced long-term (longer than 30 minutes) & short-term (less than 15 minutes) endurance capacity both in highly trained top-level endurance athletes.'[240]

A great example of this can be found in the decorated career of Peter Sagan. One of the best bike road racers in history having won the UCI Road World Championships three times, Sagan according to his coach Patxi Vila is not naturally a sprinter. Yet time and again he's won sprints and performs so well on the steep hill climbs. How? His coach claims, 'We get his speed through his strength training.' Interestingly, in the winter of 2017 *Cycling Weekly* detailed the training of Sagan and noted that most cyclists strength train in their off-season, but rarely continue once the season has started since they prefer to focus on road training (developing Specific Physical Preparedness).

But Sagan and his entire team were different and maintained an element of strength training throughout the season. This is supported by research from the *Canadian Journal of Applied Physiology* that found, 'These results suggest that strength gains can be maintained with resistance training once or twice a week while focusing on improving aerobic endurance performance without compromising the latter.'[241]

For swimming, the theory is the same but the strength/speed qualities are different.

This is all based on the SAID principle (Specific Adaptation to Imposed Demands) meaning you adapt specifically to the demands you place on your body and become very good at what you repeatedly practise. This is why 80 per cent of the training should be spent in the water and the other 20 per cent should be spent in the gym performing ancillary strength exercises that replicate the movements performed in the water, since scientists claim, 'In addition to in-water training to improve swimming performance, it can be stated that land training has positive effects on swimming.'[242]

Looking at the swim-specific dry land resistance training itself, every workout serves to:

- **Increase Propulsion.** By improving strength and speed ('added gears') in the muscles that provide propulsion in the water.
- **Reduce Drag/Resistance.** By ensuring you have the strength and endurance to maintain good body position and posture in the water.

Referring back to the figure (see below) in the *Journal of Swimming Research*, each gym session is therefore trying to positively impact on resistance and/or propulsion, two key determinants of performance.

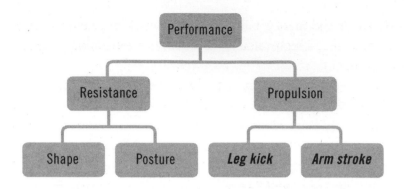

INCREASE PROPULSION: UPPER BODY

Looking at propulsion, *the Journal of Sports Medicine* stated, 'The majority of propulsive forces in swimming are produced from the upper body, with strong correlations between upper body strength and sprint performance.' Adding, 'High-velocity/force resistance-training programmes are optimal and stroke length is best achieved through resistance training with low repetitions at a high velocity/force.'[243]

This is supported by researchers who state, 'Heavy strength training on dry land (one to five repetitions maximum with pull-downs for three sets with maximal effort in the concentric phase) or sprint swimming with resistance towards propulsion (maximal pushing with the arms against fixed points or pulling a perforated bowl) may be efficient for enhanced performance, and may also possibly have positive effects on stroke mechanics.'[244]

Also, the theory is exactly the same for Alex and anyone who has impaired function of certain limbs. Research from the *Journal of Sports Medicine and Physical Fitness* found, 'Swimmers with paraplegia involved in 12 weeks' combined strength on dry land and resistance training in the water program improved strength, swimming performance and stroke parameters in comparison with swimmers training swimming alone.'[245]

So that's the theory, but how does it work in practice? How do you implement a high-velocity/force resistance-training programme for swimmers?

While we've already given examples of specific exercises along the Force-Velocity Curve, one training tool that's used to manipulate the body's speed of movement is resistance bands. Used in strength and conditioning as far back as the 1970s, resistance bands even featured in Professor Yuri Verkhoshansky's 1997 book entitled *Fundamentals of Special Strength-Training in Sport* where he detailed the way they add 'progressive' resistance to movements. What this means is, the more it's stretched the higher the resistance. This is a key characteristic that makes it very different to free weights where the resistance remains virtually the same as dictated by gravity.

This unique property of resistance bands is perhaps the main reason they've become so widely used in strength and conditioning, since experts believe the linear variable resistance provided by bands – the way it gets harder the more it's stretched – mimics what's known as the 'strength curve' of most muscles.

A 'strength curve' is a term used in kinetics.

Kinetics is the study of the body's motion, which details how a muscle's strength will change over a range of motion. Taking the commonly used bicep curl as an example, notice how you're particularly weak during the lower range of the exercise; however, as your hand (and the bar) move towards the shoulder the strength of the biceps increases.

Now, if you performed a bicep curl with a free weight you'd find you were limited in how much weight you could lift during the lowest part of the lift, your weakest point. But if you added some 'progressive resistance' in the form of a resistance band attached to the bar, you'd add more resistance at the strongest point in your range of motion, therefore adding more resistance to better stimulate strength adaptations.[246] To put it simply, you make the bicep work harder over the entire range of motion.

But the most important training adaptation for swimmers when using bands is that they improve Rate of Force Development (RFD). This is defined as the body's ability to generate the greatest amount of force in the shortest time possible. The faster your RFD the quicker and more explosive you and your movements become.

This is why research conducted at the Department of Mechanical Engineering at the University of Minnesota in Minneapolis, USA is so important. It set out to examine how the use of elastic bands in resistance training can increase performance-related parameters such as RFD. Researchers took 20 trained male volunteers and had them perform a free-weight back squat exercise with and without elastic bands. Results showed that rate of force development was significantly greater with the use of bands and concluded, 'Results indicate that there may be benefits to performing squats with elastic bands in terms of rate of force development. Practitioners concerned with improving rate of force development may want to consider incorporating this easily implemented training variation.'[247]

INCREASE PROPULSION: THE CORE

Research from the National Conditioning Association stresses a swimmer's strength training should include more than just high-velocity/force resistance-training in the upper body to improve propulsion. Instead, it must also focus on developing strength in the core to assist power and propulsion through the hips.[248] (This is all based on The Aquatic Art of 5 Limbs that we described previously). This is why it's logical that adding exercises of this nature to a swimmer's strength training programme will ultimately increase the power and speed of the stroke. The goal (thanks to the Serape Effect) is to generate power and condition the body from the inside out.[249]

One great exercise to do this is the Diagonal Downward (and Upward) Chop. Performed by holding a cable or resistance band over one shoulder, you 'chop' in a diagonal pattern past the opposite knee while focusing on fully engaging the core and serape musculature.

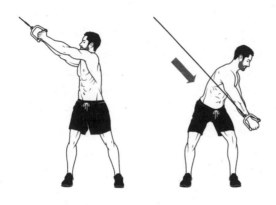

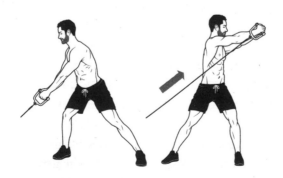

Other conditioning tools to train the Serape Effect include:

Serape Strength Exercises	Serape Strength/Speed Exercises
Turkish Get-Ups	1-arm Kettlebell Swings
1-legged Deadlifts (dumbbell held in opposing arm to the leg)	1-arm Dumbbell Snatches
	Sledge Hammer Hits
1-arm Bent Over Dumbbell Rows	Medicine Ball Side Toss
1-arm Dumbbell Chest Press	Medicine Ball Chop Throws
1-arm Suspended Rows	Medicine Ball Shotput Throws
1-arm Push-Ups	Tornado Ball Slams
1-legged Squats	Scissor Jumps
Landmine Twists	Rotational Jumps
1-leg Hip Lifts	Rotational Battle Ropes

REDUCE DRAG/RESISTANCE

As well as producing rotational power, the core also has another function. According to research from the National Conditioning Association, it plays a key role in maintaining proper posture, balance and alignment in the water. If these elements are not maintained, then resistive forces will increase and stroke technique will break down, leading to an inefficient stroke. Therefore, increasing the core strength of a swimmer will improve their ability to maintain efficient technique for the duration of the swim.

This is supported by research published in the *Journal of Sports Medicine* that found, 'The present research available supports the addition of strength training in an endurance athlete's programme for improved economy, muscle power and performance.'[250]

So how do we do this?

Put simply, we must condition the core in the gym by learning to hold, hang and balance. This is supported by research published in the *Journal of Strength and Conditioning* which wanted to, 'Evaluate the effect of unstable and unilateral exercises on core muscle activation.' Using electromyography technology, they tested the activity of the muscles in the core and found, 'The most effective means for trunk strengthening should involve back or abdominal exercises with unstable bases.' Adding, 'Furthermore, trunk strengthening can also occur when performing resistance exercises, if the exercises are performed unilaterally,' meaning with a single limb (or one side of the body).[251]

One way is to perform unilateral movements (moving one limb or one side of the body) on unstable surfaces, like a Single-Arm Swiss Ball Push-Up which creates a lot of torque through the spine, particularly in the working arm and opposite leg due to the angle of the oblique muscles and the ways our bodies stabilise from one side to the other.

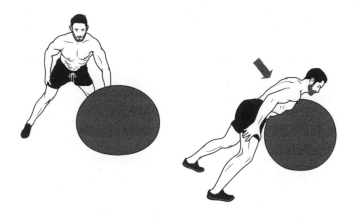

Alternatively, research from the *Journal of Human Kinetics* demonstrated that performing your push-ups (or planks) with your feet placed in gymnastic rings elicited a different kind of muscle activation in the stomach when compared to a traditional push-up on the floor. 'Therefore, suspension push-ups may be considered an advanced variation of a traditional push-up when a greater challenge is warranted.' They're not the only ones to think so either. The *Journal of Exercise Physiology* states, 'A suspension device elicited a greater activation of the stomach muscles.' Again, supporting this idea to take your planks and press-up variations off the floor and onto something less stable like an Swiss exercise ball.

That being said, unstable surface training still divides the strength and conditioning community. Research published by the National Strength and Conditioning Association stated that its 'application is still very limited'. But it is acknowledged, 'Unstable surface training has been shown to increase core muscle activity and alter neuromuscular recruitment patterns.' So, if your goal is to build a stronger core, learn to balance, alter your neuromuscular recruitment patterns by operating over a different range of motion and add some variety to your push-ups.

Next, you'll remember from the *Recovery Mesocycle* chapter that hanging (brachiating) is a lost art form and forgotten method to rehabilitate the shoulders, but it can equally serve to condition the core as well. This is based on research published by the American Association for Health, Physical Education and Recreation that studied muscle activation in the stomach during 10 strenuous abdominal exercises. What they found was, 'Intensity of contraction was greatest in the basket hang, followed by three variations of the hook sit-up.'[252] So brachiating beats the conventional sit-up in terms of muscle activation. Researchers added, 'The apparently strenuous nature of the basket hang, which is primarily a movement of thigh rather than trunk flexion, implies that this exercise may be useful in the abdominal training of highly conditioned athletes.'

BRACHIATING
Hang from a pull-up bar with your hands shoulder-width apart
Contract your lower abs and bring your knees to your chest
Twist your hips to one side in a controlled manner, keeping your chest forward at all times
Pause, then perform on the alternate side as you crunch your ribs to your hips

ROCK SOLID STRENGTH AND SPEED

To give another example, and to delve a little deeper into the strength/ speed qualities of different sports, let's look at rock climbing.

A sport that evolved from mountaineering[253] when, during the late 1800s, mountaineers became interested in climbing specific cliffs or rock formations, rock climbing quickly gained popularity and more advanced techniques and equipment were developed. This was then followed by the invention (and increased accessibility) to indoor artificial rock climbing walls which led to targeted training. Back in 2012, the *National Strength and Conditioning Journal* wrote, 'There is considerable need for the strength and conditioning professional to understand the basics of rock climbing, including its unique terminology, physiological demands, and theories for developing specialized strength training programs to enhance climbing performance and reduce the risk of climbing injuries.'

But what's meant by 'specialised strength training'?

Basically, this is about training specific muscles to perform a specific function with strength and speed qualities (on the Force-Velocity Curve) that replicate the specific conditions of the sport. Within the sport of rock climbing, no-one understands this better than Alex Honnold.

Considered the world's greatest rock climber, on 3 June 2017 he completed the first free solo climb of El Capitan in Yosemite National Park without protective equipment. Standing 3,000 ft (914 m) from base to summit, its sheer granite face was ascended by Honnold in 3 hours and 56 minutes. Bu to truly understand how he did this, you must also understand the physiological demands on the body and the different types of muscle contractions it required to complete.

SPECIFIC MUSCLE FUNCTION

Rock climbing has very precise speed and strength qualities. Firstly, it's not surprising that researchers found, 'Endurance of the shoulder girdle was substantially greater in climbers.'[254] After all, the pulling muscles (elbow flexors and shoulder extensors) are extensively used during climbing.

Equally, climbers rely heavily on their finger and wrist flexors to firmly grip holds on climbing surfaces. This is why whenever possible, climbers should modify strength training exercises to incorporate a variety of different grips. Barbells, dumbbells, and pull-up bars with large diameter handles (known as thick bars) are great training tools,[255] and another simple method is wrapping a towel around a pull-up bar to grip.[256] But to be a truly great climber, you must learn about muscle contractions and how to train them effectively.

ISOMETRIC CONTRACTIONS

This is where the muscle contracts but does not shorten, giving no movement. The plank is perhaps the best example of an isometric contraction in the gym, but when rock climbing isometric contractions are needed to stabilise the body when a climber stops to chalk one's hands, clip bolts, place gear, and contemplate his/her next move.[257] On average, 38 per cent of climbing time is spent in static positions.[258]

So, long before Alex even considered climbing El Capitan, he was incorporating climbing-specific isometric contractions into his strength training by religiously hanging from a wooden board fitted to his van (with 90 degree elbow flexion) with various finger holds to train grip over different angles.

CONCENTRIC CONTRACTIONS

This is where the muscle contracts and shortens in length. The upward movement of a bicep curl is a simple example of a concentric contraction in the bicep, but with rock climbing it becomes more complex since it's a sport that requires so many whole-body power movements. The best example of a quick and powerful movement performed during climbing is the dyno, a movement where a climber literally leaps off the climbing surface in attempt to reach a hold otherwise unattainable. The dyno requires considerable activation of various ankle, knee and hip extensor muscles to produce a large amount of force in a short time, sufficient to maximise vertical acceleration.

To train for movements like this, exercises like the hang clean, box jumps, muscle-ups and plyometric training as a whole should be included within an athlete's programme. Looking at the Force-Velocity Curve, it conditions the muscles to work within the *Peak Power Zone* and *Speed-Strength Zone*. Specifically, for climbers, bouldering also offers a great way to train at this end of the force-velocity while also drilling technique and developing sports specific preparedness.

ECCENTRIC CONTRACTIONS

This is where the muscle is in tension while it lengthens. A good example is the downward movement of a dumbbell in a biceps curl. Or when you land on two feet from a jump and bend your knees, you'll notice the quadriceps are in tension to cushion the impact, but are lengthening. Eccentric contractions are also an integral component of rock climbing. When a climber loses contact with a hold (e.g. removing one hand from the surface in attempt to reach the next hold) various upper-body muscles may contract eccentrically to maintain joint stability and control his/her position to the wall. Or if a climber must climb down a particular route, they must rely on controlled eccentric contractions to lower the body, essentially climbing the route in reverse.

DYNAMIC STRENGTH INDEX

When designing a strength routine for an adventure, just as important as your adventure's strength and speed qualities is your Dynamic Strength Index (DSI).[259] Also known as the Dynamic Strength Deficit[260] or the Explosive Strength Deficit,[261] this is simply the difference between an athlete's maximal strength and their ballistic strength. Or, put more simply, the difference between an athlete's 1RM back-squat and their standing vertical jump.

The reason this is so important is because:

Maximal Strength/Force. Measures an athlete's ability to produce maximum force during a concentric/isometric exercise.

- *How to Test:* This can be measured through a 1RM back-squat. But more recently sports scientists have preferred an isometric mid-thigh pull. This is where an athlete stands on the force plate gripping the bar as they would to perform a deadlift with knees and hips flexed, back straight and head up. The height of the barbell is adjusted so that it crosses the thighs at the midpoint between the hip and knee joints. When instructed the athlete pulls upward on the bar rapidly with maximal effort, maintaining the effort until the force output starts to decline.

But strength within sport and adventure usually has a speed component too, whether that's Alex Honnold performing a dyno during a rock climb or an MMA athlete performing a judo throw to take his opponent to the floor. This is why we need to measure:

Ballistic Strength/Force. Measures an athlete's ability to produce force at speed during a ballistic (fast) exercise in a short timeframe.

- *How to Test*: This can be measured by having the athlete perform a countermovement vertical jump. This is where they start from an upright standing position, make a preliminary downward movement by flexing at the knees and hips, then immediately extend the knees and hips again to jump vertically.

Looking back at the Force-Velocity Curve, the DSI essentially measures an athlete's ability to operate optimally along all parts of the curve.[262] Knowing this is so important when designing an effective periodised training plan, since it allows the coach to identify how forceful (i.e. strong) the athlete is and how much of that strength they can use during high-speed ballistic movements.[263]

So that's the theory. Now delving more into the detail, this is how you calculate your DSI and how it will have a profound impact on your periodised programme for the week, month and year.

THE MATHS: MEASURING DYNAMIC STRENGTH INDEX

With force measured in newtons (N), the equation looks like this:

Dynamic Strength Index = Ballistic Peak Force (N)/Maximal (Isometric) Force (N)

Comparing the Countermovement Jump (CMJ) and Isometric Mid-Thigh Pull (IMTP) of three different athletes, their DSI scores would look like this:

- **ATHLETE A:** 1,450 (N)/3,178 (N) = 0.46 (46 per cent)
- **ATHLETE A:** 2,500 (N)/3,000 (N) = 0.83 (83 per cent)
- **ATHLETE C:** 2,600 (N)/2,600 (N) = 1 (100 per cent)

This can be represented in a table as shown.

Exercise	CMJ Peak Force (N)	IMTP Peak Force (N)	DSI
Athlete A	1,450	3,178	0.46 (46%)
Athlete B	2,500	3,000	0.83 (83%)
Athlete C	2,600	2,600	1 (100%)

The DSI score reflects the percentage of their 'force potential' that's not being used during fast, ballistic movements (like a countermovement jump).[264] Therefore, theoretically speaking, if an athlete can register a DSI score of 1 (like athlete C), they are capable of using their full 'force potential' during a fast, explosive, ballistic exercise. In contrast, if an athlete has a low DSI score (like athlete A) they are less capable of utilising their 'force potential' during a fast, explosive, ballistic exercise.

In summary:

- A smaller DSI score means more time should be spent training within the Peak Power Training Zone and Speed-Strength Training Zone of the Force-Velocity Curve to become a better athlete.[265]
- A higher DSI score means more time should be spent on developing maximal strength (i.e. force production) training within the Maximum Strength Training Zone and Strength-Speed Training Zone of the Force-Velocity Curve to become a more well-rounded athlete.[266]

Score	DSI Score	Training Emphasis Recommendation
Low	<0.60	SPEED-STRENGTH TRAINING ZONE
Moderate	0.60–0.80	ZONES ACROSS THE FORCE-VELOCITY CURVE
High	>0.80	MAXIMUM STRENGTH TRAINING ZONE

The Dynamic Strength Index is one of the most underrated metrics in athletic performance, and understanding it will have a profound impact on your training.

As for me, I continued to train in secret away from the team. I understood the strength and speed qualities of my adventure, my need for more 'gears' and my Dynamic Strength Index, which is why the strength sessions for my *Build Mesocycle* contained a blend of different training zones from the Force-Velocity Curve.

BUILD TRAINING PLAN (SPRING): MICROCYCLE (WEEK'S PLAN)

SPEED, STRENGTH & SPORT SPECIFIC: THE FORMAT

The entire focus of this mesocycle is to develop *Specific Physical Preparedness*. Importantly, once the exact details of your adventure have been identified (and you have checked into 'fight camp') you must be so strict with your strength and conditioning. Put simply, if any session, exercise or training tool doesn't contribute to your overall goal, you need to eliminate it from your *Build Mesocycle* since now is the time to specialise (hence running no longer features within any of our training).

This is (again) all based on the SAID principle, meaning you adapt specifically to the demands you place on your body and become very good at what you repeatedly practise. Hence, why 80 per cent of the training is now spent in the water and the other 20 per cent is now spent in the gym replicating the movements in the water.

Deciding to keep the same format/split routine of the strength and conditioning sessions, they remain biomechanically divided and are kept very short. Since the goal of the strength sessions is now less focused on work capacity, but instead it's to improve your Dynamic Strength Index. Indeed, research published in *the Journal of Sports Medicine* entitled 'Exercise-training intervention studies in competitive swimming' found that, 'High training volumes do not pose any immediate advantage over lower volumes (with higher intensity) for swim performance.'[267]

The same is also true of the high-intensity (anaerobic) interval sessions, where the goal is to operate at a higher intensity, for a short time and with enough recovery between sessions due to the demands it places on the body. On this note, many coaches recommend that high-intensity interval training (HIIT) sessions are separated by at least 48 hours.[268] So, as the intensity of this mesocycle increases (yet volume decreases) the microcycle contains nine sessions per week which consists of:

- THREE strength (and speed) sessions operating within the Force-Velocity Curve.
- THREE slow and long (10 km) open water swims operating in Zone 2 to continue building a solid aerobic base ('gas tank') while also developing Specific Physical Preparedness.
- THREE high-intensity interval sessions operating in Zones 4 and 5 to improve anaerobic fitness (add some 'jet engine afterburners' to the already sizeable 'gas tank').

Also now, more than ever, the scheduling of the sessions is so important. This is because during your *Build Mesocycle* the intensity is increased, so (again) your recovery is on a 'knife edge', meaning when there is no training session planned you must consciously activate your parasympathetic nervous system and continue to prioritise sleep.

But the other reason it's so important to schedule (and separate) your workouts is because during a training week (microcycle) you're now trying to elicit more physiological adaptations within the body, whether that's speed and strength in the gym, anaerobic fitness in the pool or aerobic fitness in the lake. Therefore, without proper scheduling and sufficient rest there is a greater danger of 'diluting the potency' of the training, not sending a clear cellular signal' to the body and unfortunately falling victim to the 'interference phenomenon'.

Fortunately, if you consider your macrocycle in its entirety, you understand it is possible to adapt to multiple workouts in a single day, if:

- You separate your workouts enough within the microcycle (day and week).

- You have a high enough work capacity (built through the *Base Mesocycle*).

Finally, you'll notice strength-based rehab has been reintroduced to the workouts. When researchers monitored, 'The average competitive swimmer swims approximately 60,000 metres to 80,000 metres per week. With a typical count of 8 to 10 strokes per 25-m lap, each shoulder performs 30 000 rotations each week,' they found that, 'This places tremendous stress on the shoulder girdle musculature and glenohumeral joint and is why shoulder pain is the most frequent musculoskeletal complaint among competitive swimmers.'[269]

The good news is that studies show that by training the lesser-used shoulder muscles[270] you can combat these imbalances, restore the natural structure within the shoulder girdle musculature[271] and prevent any imbalances and overuse injuries.[272] Therefore, ensuring the body is bulletproof[273] and able to cope with the increased intensity of the *Build Mesocycle*.[274]

All of this represented in a table in which a week's training looks like this:

	Monday	Tuesday	Wednesday	Thursday	Friday	Saturday	Sunday
MORNING	Swim Interval Training	Swim 10 km Open Water	Swim Interval Training	Swim 10 km Open Water	Swim Interval Training	Swim 10 km Open Water	REST
PURPOSE	Anaerobic Fitness (Zones 4 & 5)	Aerobic Fitness (Zone 2)	Anaerobic Fitness (Zones 4 & 5)	Aerobic Fitness (Zone 2)	Anaerobic Fitness (Zones 4 & 5)	Aerobic Fitness (Zone 2)	
AFTERNOON	'Pull' Routine		Lower Body Routine		'Push' Routine		
PURPOSE	Supplementary Strength and Speed Training		Supplementary Strength and Speed Training		Supplementary Strength and Speed Training		

6-DAY BASE PROGRAMME

MONDAY & FRIDAY

AEROBIC FITNESS: 10 KM SWIM (ZONE 2)

Exercises	Time	Distance	Intensity
Swim	120+ minutes	10 km	Zone 2 60–70 per cent of your maximum heart rate

Coaching Cues

These sessions operate in Zone 2 to continue building a solid aerobic base and 'gas tank' (your heart, lungs and cardiorespiratory system) while also developing Specific Physical Preparedness and swimming technique focusing on body position, breathing, arm stroke and leg kick.

ANAEROBIC FITNESS: HIGH-INTENSITY INTERVALS (ZONES 4 AND 5)

Exercises	Intervals	Time	Distance	Intensity
WARM-UP	1 km	15–20 minutes	1 km	Zone 2 60–70 per cent of your maximum heart rate

Coaching Cues

The purpose of the warm-up is to acclimatise to the cold water (if being performed in a lake or the sea) and to help prepare the body for the session ahead by raising your body temperature and increasing blood flow to your muscles.

Exercises	Intervals	Time	Distance	Intensity
TECHNIQUE	10 x 200 m	30–40 minutes	2km	Zone 3 70–80 per cent of your maximum heart rate

Coaching Cues

The primary goal here to begin developing Specific Physical Preparedness by drilling an efficient technique at a faster pace. Focusing specifically on body position, breathing, arm stroke and leg kick.

Exercises	Intervals	Time	Distance	Intensity
MAIN SET	10 x 200 m	30 minutes	2 km	Zones 4 and 5 80–100 per cent of your maximum heart rate

Coaching Cues

This is the most important part of the entire session. This is where oxygen use increases, heart rate elevates, fuel is burnt, chemicals build up which contribute to exhaustion, water is lost, heat accumulates, muscles fatigue and the molecular energy of the muscles (adenosine triphosphate) runs low. But finishing this will ensure you improve your anaerobic fitness ('jet engine afterburners') and improve the buffering-capacity of your muscles to cope with fatigue

Exercises	Intervals	Time	Distance	Intensity
COOL-DOWN	500 m	10 minutes	500 m	Zones 1 and 2 50–70 per cent of your maximum heart rate

Coaching Cues

The goal of a cool-down is to reduce heart and breathing rates, gradually cool body temperature, return muscles to their optimal length-tension relationships and restore physiologic systems close to baseline as you prepare to 'switch on' the parasympathetic nervous system and begin the recovery process.

MONDAY: 'PULL' TRAINING

SUPPLEMENTARY STRENGTH AND SPEED TRAINING

Exercises	Repetitions	Sets	Rest	Physiological Adaptation
Passive Hang (Brachiating) (p 301)	60 seconds	3	90 seconds	Strength Rehab/ Prehab
Scapula Pull-Ups (p 302)	10	3	90 seconds	Strength Rehab/ Prehab
Overhead Medicine Ball Slams (p 303)	4–6	3	90 seconds	Speed Strength Training Zone
Overhand (pronated) Weighted Pull-Ups (p 303)	8–10	3	90 seconds	Strength-Speed Training Zone
Hanging Barbell High Pull (p 307)	4–6	3	90 seconds	Peak Power Training
Band-Resisted Single Arm Rows (p 309)	4–6	3	90 seconds	Peak Power Training
Cable Face Pulls (p 308)	10–12	3	60 seconds	Strength Rehab/ Prehab
Single-Arm Plank Rope Pulls (p 310)	60 seconds (each arm) or 20 metres	4	60 seconds	Strength/ Endurance & Work Capacity

WEDNESDAY: LOWER BODY ROUTINE

SUPPLEMENTARY STRENGTH AND SPEED TRAINING

Exercises	Repetitions	Sets	Rest	Physiological Adaptation
Box Jumps (p 315)	5–7	3	120 seconds	Speed Strength Training Zone
Front Seated Squats (p 311)	8–10	3	90 seconds	Strength Training Zone
Single-Arm Dumbbell Side Lunge and Touch (p 316)	10 (each side)	3	90 seconds	Stability Strength, Posture and Body Position
Battle Rope Wrestler Throws (p 317)	8 (each side)	3	90 seconds	Speed Strength Training Zone
The Stability Ball Log Roll (p 317)	60 seconds	3	90 seconds	Stability Strength, Posture and Body Position
Pallof Hold and Press (p 318)	60 seconds	3	90 seconds	Stability Strength, Posture and Body Position
V-Sit Flutter Kick (p 318)	60 seconds	3	90 seconds	Stability Strength, Posture and Body Position

FRIDAY: 'PUSH' TRAINING

SUPPLEMENTARY STRENGTH AND SPEED TRAINING

Exercises	Repetitions	Sets	Rest	Physiological Adaptation
External Rotation with Band (p 320)	8–12	3	90 seconds	Strength Rehab/Prehab
Internal Rotation with Band (p 320)	8–12	3	90 seconds	Strength Rehab/Prehab
Scapula Push-Ups (p 319)	10	3	90 seconds	Strength Rehab/Prehab
Plyometric Push-Ups (p 321)	5	3	90 seconds	Speed Strength Training Zone
Band-Resisted Push-Ups (p 321)	8–10	3	90 seconds	Strength Training Zone
Single-Arm Kettlebell Shoulder Press (p 323)	12 (each arm)	3	60 seconds	Strength Rehab/Prehab
Band-Resisted Tricep Push-Downs (p 325)	12	3	60 seconds	Peak Power Training Zone
Battle Rope Plank Single-Arm Waves (p 326)	60 seconds (each arm)	4	60 seconds	Strength/Endurance & Work Capacity

18-WEEK MARATHON GUIDE | TRAINING NOTES

As another example, the 18-week marathon training guide on the following page puts all the above theory into practice for someone who wants to use the solid aerobic base ('gas tank' conditioned through Zone 2 training at 60 to 70 per cent of their maximum heart rate) that they built during the Base Mesocycle to now specialise in long-distance running. To do this they must now prioritise running (Specific Physical Preparedness) and condition the body to work more efficiently at high intensities (adding 'jet engine afterburners' where you operate above your anaerobic threshold) by manipulating the intensity and volume of the training. With this said, the keys to this program are:

- All units are listed in kilometres
- The hardest and most intense training period is between weeks 8 to 15
- Numbers that are in brackets indicate the run should be done at a pace higher than your anaerobic threshold pace
- Numbers underlined indicate you should run at race pace
- The final long-distance run should be done 2 weeks prior to the race.
- 2 days before the race, jog 2-3 km and increase speed over 1km to simulate the race and stimulate the legs

		Monday	Tuesday	Wednesday	Thursday	Friday	Saturday	Sunday	Distance per week
Week 1	Jog at a slow and comfortable pace (zone 2)	Rest	3 km	3 km	3 km	Rest	3 km	Rest	12 km
Week 2		Rest	3 km	3 km	3 km	Rest	5 km	Rest	14 km
Week 3	Run above your anaerobic threshold pace twice per week	Rest	5 km	Rest	5 km	Rest	5 km	Rest	15 km
Week 4		Rest	5 km	5 km	5 km	Rest	5 km	Rest	20 km
Week 5	Run faster than your anaerobic threshold pace twice a week.	Rest	(5 km)	Rest	(5 km)	Rest	10 km	Rest	20 km
Week 6		Rest	(7 km)	Rest	(7 km)	Rest	10 km	Rest	24 km
Week 7	Perform a long-distance run on Sat/ Sun that is slower than anaerobic threshold pace.	Rest	(7 km)	Rest	(7 km)	Rest	12 km	Rest	26 km
Week 8		Rest	(7 km)	Rest	(7 km)	Rest	15 km	Rest	29 km
Week 9		Rest	(7 km)	Rest	5 km	Rest	15 km	Rest	27 km
Week 10	Run faster than your anaerobic threshold pace once a week.	Rest	5 km	(10 km)	Rest	Rest	20 km	Rest	35 km
Week 11		Rest	5 km	(10 km)	Rest	Rest	25 km	Rest	40 km
Week 12	Perform a long-distance run on Sat/ Sun that is slower than anaerobic threshold pace.	Rest	5 km	(10 km)	Rest	Rest	15 km	Rest	30 km
Week 13		Rest	5 km	(10 km)	Rest	5 km	25 km	Rest	45 km
Week 14	On the other days jog at a slow and comfortable pace	Rest	5 km	(10 km)	Rest	Rest	15 km	Rest	30 km
Week 15		Rest	5 km	(10 km)	Rest	5 km	30 km	Rest	50 km
Week 16	Run at race pace but be sure to avoid overtraining as the intensity increases to match 'race pace'	Rest	Rest	5 km	10 km	Rest	15 km	Rest	30 km
Week 17		Rest	7 km	Rest	5 km	Rest	5 km	Rest	17 km
Week 18		Rest	5 km	Rest	3 km	(1 km)	Rest	RACE	9 km

12-WEEK (OLYMPIC DISTANCE) TRIATHLON GUIDE | TRAINING NOTES

To give you one more example, turn the page for a template training plan for an Olympic-distance triathlon that consists of a 1.5km swim, 40km bike ride and 10km run. The reason I love this particular program is because you essentially have 3 different sports to specialise in which highlights just how important it is to develop an 'athletic base' and work capacity (in your Base Mesocycle) beforehand to tolerate multiple sessions. Again, you simply can't go from 5 hours training per week (during the Recovery Mesocycle) to 20+ hours per week (like most elite Ironman triathletes) since it will be too much stress for the body to handle.

Now it's important to first note that every athlete is different, but generally speaking the average triathlete spends about 20% of the total race time swimming, 50% cycling and about 30% running. Which is why most coaches would recommend your training match these splits. What this means is you do an equal number of swim, bike and run workouts, but your swimming workouts should be shorter than run and your run shorter than your bike.

To put this into an example, if you train 6 times per week, you will swim, bike and run twice but your longest bike ride might be one hour, whereas your swims last 30 minutes each and your runs, 40 minutes. You then increase this 'workload' incrementally throughout the time you have available before your race, making sure you allow yourself enough time to recover. This is the basic theory that governs the 12-week plan.

	Monday	Tuesday	Wednesday	Thursday	Friday	Saturday	Sunday
Week 1	**Swimming Specific** - 10 minutes warm-up - 10 x 25m drills with 20 seconds rest - 10 x 50m (25m hard/25m easy) with 20 seconds rest - 5 minutes warm down	**Running Specific** - 10 minutes warm-up - 6 x 20 seconds hill reps and jog down recovery - 15 minutes running at 80% Max. Heart Rate - 5 minutes warm down **Strength session.** 30 minutes	**Rest**	**Cycling Specific** Turbo 40 minutes. (10 minutes warm-up. 10 x 60 seconds high cadence (low gear at <75% Max. Heart Rate) and 60 seconds easy. 10 minutes warm down)	**Swimming Specific** 30-45 minutes technique work	**Running Specific** 40 minutes easy and off-road **Strength session.** 30 minutes	**Cycling Specific** 60 minutes steady pace
Week 2	**Swimming Specific** -10 minutes warm-up; - 10 x 25m drills with 20 seconds rest - 15 x 50m (25m hard/25m easy) with 20 seconds res; - 5 minutes warm down	**Running Specific** - 10 minutes warm-up - 8 x 20 seconds hill reps and jog down recovery - 15 minutes running at 80% Max. Heart Rate - 5 minutes warm down **Strength session.** 30 minutes	**Rest**	**Cycling Specific** Turbo 45 minutes, (10 minutes warm-up. 12 x 60 seconds high cadence (low gear at <75% Max. Heart Rate) and 60 seconds easy. 10 minutes warm down)	**Swimming Specific** 30-45 minutes technique work	**Running Specific** 45 minutes easy and off-road **Strength session.** 30 minutes	**Cycling Specific** 70 minutes steady pace

	Swimming Specific	Running Specific	Rest	Cycling Specific	Swimming Specific	Running Specific	Cycling Specific
Week 3	10 minutes warm-up; 10 x 25m drills with 20 seconds rest; 20 x 50m (25m hard/25m easy) with 20 seconds rest; 5 minutes warm down	- 10 minutes warm-up - 10 x 20 seconds hill reps with jog down recovery - 15 minutes running at 80% Max. Heart Rate - 5 minutes warm down **Strength session.** 30 minutes	Rest	Turbo 40 minutes, (10 seconds warm-up, 15 x 60 seconds high cadence (low gear at <75% Max. Heart Rate) and 60 seconds easy. 10 minutes warm down)	30-45 minutes technique work	50 minutes easy and off-road **Strength session.** 30 minutes	80 minutes steady pace
Week 4	Complete 50% of race distance non-stop	- 10 minutes warm-up - 15 x 20 seconds brisk strides at 5k pace and 40 seconds recovery - 5 minutes warm down **Weights.** 30 minutes	Rest	25 minutes turbo. 10 minutes warm-up, 10 x 30 seconds at high cadence (low gear at <75% Max. Heart Rate) and 30 seconds recovery. 5 minutes warm down	30 minutes technique work	30 minutes easy and off-road **Strength session.** 30 minutes	45 minutes steady pace

(continued)

	Monday	Tuesday	Wednesday	Thursday	Friday	Saturday	Sunday
Week 5	**Swimming Specific** - 10 minutes warm-up - 10 x 25m drills with 20 seconds rest - 10 x 100m (50m hard/ 50m easy) with 20 seconds rest - 5 minute warm down	**Running Specific** - 10 minutes warm-up - 6 x 30 seconds hill reps with jog down recovery - 15 seconds running at 80-85% Max. Heart Rate - 5 minutes warm down. **Strength session.** 30 minutes	Rest	**Cycling Specific** Turbo 40 minutes (10 minutes warm-up; 10 x 30 seconds at max intensity; 90 seconds easy; 10 minutes warm down)	**Swimming Specific** 45-60 minutes technique and endurance work	**Running Specific** 45 minutes easy and off-road. Find a hilly route to build leg strength	**Cycling Specific** 70 minutes hilly at steady pace. Stay seated on hills to build leg strength
Week 6	**Swimming Specific** - 10 minutes warm-up; - 10 x 25m drills with 20 seconds rest; - 15 x 50m (25m hard/25m easy) with 20 seconds rest - 5 minutes warm down	**Running Specific** - 10 minutes warm-up - 8 x 20 seconds hill reps and jog down recovery - 15 seconds running at 80% Max. Heart Rate - 5 minutes warm down **Strength session.** 30 minutes	Rest	**Cycling Specific** Turbo 45 minutes, (10 minutes warm-up. 12 x 60 seconds high cadence (low gear at <75% Max. Heart Rate) and 60 seconds easy. 10 minutes warm down)	**Swimming Specific** 30-45 minutes technique work	**Running Specific** 45 minutes easy and off-road. **Strength session.** 30 minutes	**Cycling Specific** 70 minutes steady pace

	Swimming Specific	Running Specific	Rest	Cycling Specific	Swimming Specific	Running Specific	Cycling Specific
Week 7	**Swimming Specific** - 10 minutes warm-up - 10 x 25m drills with 20 seconds rest - 20 x 50m (25m hard/25m easy) with 20 seconds rest - 5 minutes warm down	**Running Specific** - 10 minutes warm-up - 10 x 20 seconds hill reps with jog down recovery - 15 minutes running at 80% Max. Heart Rate - 5 minutes warm down **Strength session.** 30 minutes	**Rest**	**Cycling Specific** Turbo 40 minutes, (10 seconds warm-up, 15 x 60 seconds high cadence (low gear at <75% Max. Heart Rate) and 60 seconds easy. 10 minutes warm down)	**Swimming Specific** 30-45 minutes technique work	**Running Specific** 50 minutes easy and off-road **Strength session.** 30 minutes	**Cycling Specific** 80 minutes steady pace
Week 8	**Swimming Specific** Complete 50% of race distance non-stop	**Running Specific** - 10 minutes warm-up - 15 x 20 seconds brisk strides at 5k pace and 40 seconds recovery - 5 minutes warm down **Strength session.** 30 minutes	**Rest**	**Cycling Specific** 25 minutes turbo. 10 minutes warm-up, 10 x 30 seconds at high cadence (low gear <75% Max. Heart Rate) and 30 seconds recovery. 5 minutes warm down	**Swimming Specific** 30 minutes technique work	**Running Specific** 30 minutes easy and off-road **Strength session.** 30 minutes	**Cycling Specific** 45 minutes steady pace

(continued)

	Monday	Tuesday	Wednesday	Thursday	Friday	Saturday	Sunday
Week 9	**Swimming Specific** -10 minutes warm-up. - 10 x 25m drills with 20 seconds rest - 6 x -100m hard with 30 seconds rest. - 5 minutes warm down	**Running Specific** - 10 minutes warm-up - 6 x 30 seconds hill reps and jog down recovery - 2 x 5 minutes running at 85-90% Max. Heart Rate + 2 minutes active recovery. - 5 minutes warm down. **Strength session.** 30 minutes	**Rest**	**Cycling Specific** Turbo 45 minutes (10 minutes warm-up, 8 x 2 minutes at 85-90% Max. Heart Rate and 60 seconds easy spin with 10 minutes cool down) 5 minutes run off the bike	**Swimming Specific** 45-60 minutes, open water if possible. If not, include open-water skills	**Running Specific** 55 minutes off road and easy. Run on terrain similar to race route. **Strength session.** 30 minutes	**Cycling Specific** 70 minutes including 10 minutes at goal race pace
Week 10	**Swimming Specific** - 10 minutes warm-up - 10 x 25m drills with 20 seconds rest - 8 x 100m hard with 30 seconds rest after each 100m. - 5 minutes cool down	**Running Specific** - 10 minutes warm-up - 8 x 30 seconds hill reps and jog down recovery - 2 x 8 minutes running at 85-90% Max. Heart Rate with 2 minutes active recovery. - 5 minutes cool down. **Strength session.** 30 minutes	**Rest**	**Cycling Specific** Turbo 45 minutes (10 minutes warm-up, 5 x 3 minutes at 85-90% MAX. Heart Rate with 90 seconds easy spin and 10 minutes cool down) 10 minutes run off the bike	**Swimming Specific** 45-60 minutes open water if possible. If not, include open-water skills	**Running Specific** 55 minutes off road and easy. Run on terrain similar to race route. **Strength session.** 30 minutes	**Cycling Specific** 80 minutes including 15 minutes at goal race pace

Week 11	**Swimming Specific**	**Running Specific**	**Rest**	**Cycling Specific**	**Swimming Specific**	**Running Specific**	**Cycling Specific**
	- 10 minutes warm-up - 10 x 25m drills with 20 seconds rest - 10 x 100m hard + 30 seconds rest - 5 minutes cool down	- 10 minutes warm-up. - 10 x 30 seconds hill reps and jog down recovery. - 15 minutes running at 85-90% Max. Heart Rate - 5 minutes cool down **Strength session.** 30 minutes		Turbo 45 minutes. 10 minutes warm-up, 3 x 5 minutes at 85-90%MHR and 2 minutes easy spin. 10 minutes cool down and 15 minutes run off the bike	45-60 minutes open water if possible. If not, include open-water skills	40 minutes off road. Run on terrain similar to race route. **Strength session.** 30 minutes	90 minutes including mid 20 minutes goal race pace
Week 12	**Swimming Specific**	**Rest**	**Cycling Specific**	**Rest**	**Swimming Specific**	**Cycling Specific**	**Race**
	- 10 minutes warm-up - 10 x 50m drills with 20 seconds rest - 6 x 50m sprints at goal race pace and 30 seconds rest - 5 minutes easy cool down		**Cycling Specific** - 15 minutes warm-up - 15 minutes sustained effort at goal race pace. **Running Specific** - 5 minutes at goal race pace and 5 minutes easy jog to cool down		**Swimming Specific** 15 minutes including 5 x 25-50m sprints	**Cycling Specific** 15 minutes including middle 5 minutes at goal race pace. **Running Specific** 5 minutes easy pace off the bike	

SUMMER | PEAK
MESOCYCLE OVERVIEW

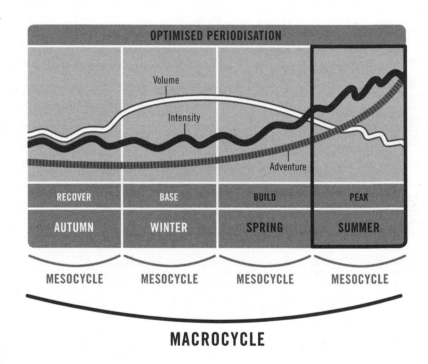

YOUR MOST POWERFUL WEAPON IS A RESOLUTE REFUSAL TO QUIT

After swimming many miles in many lakes, our *Build Mesocycle* was complete.

Yet despite our progress, I was still nervous. As an athlete I continued to train in secret and prepare for a Channel relay swim I hoped I'd never have to join. Then as a coach I watched on, session after session, praying and hoping the team's aerobic fitness ('gas tank') was now complemented by an enhanced anaerobic system ('jet engine afterburners') and would work in synergy with their enhanced speed and strength ('additional gears').

If these improvements had been made . . . we stood a chance.

If they hadn't . . . we were out of time.

Because once you reach the *Peak Mesocycle* part of the macrocycle (year) most physiologically adaptations in strength, speed and stamina *need* to have already occurred within the body after systematically and scientifically building them throughout the year. Too many coaches, athletes and adventurers don't understand this, but if you're trying to get faster, fitter and stronger at this stage of the macrocycle (year) it's too late and your adventure may be doomed to fail. Instead, during the *Peak Mesocycle* the focus should be on *maintaining* strength, speed and stamina while really beginning to focus on:

- **Refining Skills.** This is where technique is tweaked and performance is perfected, as any modifications that can be made to further develop Specific Physical Preparedness are studied and implemented.
- **Replicating & Rehearsing 'Race Conditions'.** Finding terrain and an environment that serves to mimic the conditions of the adventure. For us this meant finding water, waves and weather that we'd come to experience in the English Channel.
- **Honestly Asking Yourself if You're Ready.** This final point is so important, but also the hardest to implement. This is because after an entire year of training, you might not be ready, according to studies in sports science and human genetics.

- **The Power of the 1 per cent.** This is a doctrine of marginal gains and based on the premise that small incremental improvements (even just 1 per cent) in any process (physical, mental or technological) will eventually add up to a significant improvement when they are all added together.
- **Plank to Peak.** Towards the end of the *Peak Mesocycle* (as you prepare to embark on your adventure) the intensity of the training remains high, but the volume of training drops dramatically to ensure you're not overtrained before even beginning.

After some of the team were 'spooked' by the phantom tide of Lake Windermere, I needed them to experience a real tide as we begun replicating and rehearsing 'race conditions' and they graduated from the lake to the sea. Which is why, addressing all of the above, I took the team to Burgh Island.

STARTING THE PEAK MESOCYCLE
SUMMER 2019, BURGH ISLAND, ENGLAND

It was 2 June 2019 as I stood on the cliffs looking out to Burgh Island. An iconic landmark on the coast of south Devon, it sits about 250 metres from the mainland and is famous for the luxury Burgh Island Hotel that was built in 1929 and has welcomed many high-profile guests over the years, from Winston Churchill to Agatha Christie and The Beatles, to enjoy the stunning scenery and hotel's unique art deco interior.

But I hadn't brought the team here for a history lesson or the art.

No, the reason I had brought them here was to experience a *real* tide while swimming at sea. A unique feature of Burgh Island is the way in which it is only accessible by foot during low tide. During high tide when sea levels rise, the sandy causeway that connects the mainland to the island disappears under the water and can only be reached by boarding the 'sea tractor' that has been ferrying visitors back and forth since 1969. Like clockwork, this process is then repeated (approximately) every six hours.

Standing on the cliffs looking out to sea with the team, this was essentially the perfect 'swimming pool' for today's session, as they would begin to learn how the sea can (and so often will) push, pull and bully you if you let it and don't apply all you've learned in training.

But before we tackled the open sea, I needed the team to graduate from the lagoon. Owned and managed by the Burgh Island Hotel, the lagoon is a natural seawater bathing pool that's 20 metres wide and 50 metres in length, surrounded by rocks and 30 ft cliffs that offer complete privacy for those swimming. Filled with water directly from the English Channel, this would be ideal to replicate 'race conditions' since the temperature, visibility, buoyancy and salinity (saltiness) of the water would be identical to the conditions they would find when swimming to France.

For some members of the team, they welcomed the chance to acclimatise and become accustomed to the new conditions. For others, the assault of the saltwater on their tongues was another form of askēsis (and eustress) that they would rather do without.

'My tongue feels furry,' Linford said, stopping five minutes into the warm-up.

I couldn't help but laugh.

He was 6 ft 2 in (188 cm) tall and, although 27 years on from his Olympic gold in 1992, he still possessed the musculature of a prize-winning racehorse. But every superhero has a weakness and it seemed Linford's was an aversion to seaweed, saltwater and anything found floating in the sea.

'Ok, what's that?' he asked concerned, pointing at the water.

'Sea foam,' I replied.

I then explained how it forms when dissolved organic matter in the ocean is churned up. What that 'organic matter' is exactly usually depends on what part of the coast you are on, but it's likely this particular sea foam could be from large blooms of algae that had decayed offshore. Visibly grimacing and wincing, I could see Linford wasn't overjoyed at the idea of sharing his swimming pool with decaying algae.

'Think of it like a cold, salty bubble bath,' I said.

Far from happy, Linford reluctantly got back into the water. Not because he wanted to, but because as a coach and athlete he knew he had to, since replicating 'race conditions' was a necessary part of the *Peak Mesocycle*.

After another 30 minutes, I saw other members of the team begin to struggle with their tastebuds too. Stopping during a slow, low-intensity, aerobic session, Rachel emerged from the lagoon trying to spit the sea foam from her mouth.

'Can I get a bottle of water?' she asked.

'No,' I replied sternly. 'Give me an hour of unbroken swimming and I'll give you a bottle of water.'

Watching as she headed back into the lagoon to finish the session, I will be honest, I felt bad. Rachel had always been nervous of the sea, but as a mum she didn't want to pass this same fear onto her daughter and so wanted to embark on this particular aquatic adventurer to change her family's 'relationship' with the water. It was a truly noble reason to be swimming, which made administering tough love harder.

But the reality was we needed to begin rehearsing and mimicking the conditions of the adventure in water, waves and weather that we'd come to experience in the English Channel. As a relay, that meant the team would be swimming in hour-long intervals with no food, rest or water. If they stopped in the Channel for a bottle of water, they'd be completely at the mercy of the sea and risk being pushed back.

An hour passed and tongues had been suitably trained and tested, which meant it was time for the team to wash the decaying algae sea foam from their mouths and visit the Burgh Island Hotel restaurant for dinner as we waited for high tide. I then informed the team that once this arrived, and the sandy causeway connecting the island to the mainland was underwater, their second session would begin and they'd swim back to the mainland for their first maiden voyage at sea.

Not surprisingly, the selection of sandwiches served for dinner that day were accompanied by a barrage of questions from the team. Everyone was keen to know what lay in the water waiting for them that afternoon.

'Are there jellyfish?' Wes asked.

'Do I need to be worried about the waves?' Tessa asked.

'Has anyone ever died trying the swim from the island to mainland?' Sair asked.

I stopped and put down my tuna sandwich and then looked them all in the eyes. As their coach (and friend) I couldn't and wouldn't lie to them. It was very important that they realised the dangers of sea swimming and the severity of underestimating the ocean.

'Yes, is the answer to all your questions,' I replied.

Silence surrounded the table. The safety and security of Tinside Lido in Plymouth were now a distant memory, and the delicate waves caused by passing boats in Lake Windermere (along with the phantom tide) now seemed so tame.

Checking my watch and the tidal charts, I then announced the second session, and swim back to the mainland, would begin in two hours. Gathering around the table the team then asked how best to mentally prepare for their first sea swim. I considered my response carefully.

'Have you ever heard the expression, "Prepare for war, but pray for peace?"' I said.

'Yes,' the team collectively replied.

'Well, my advice would be leave Burgh Island praying for calm seas and favourable winds, but prepare to get a "wet willy" from a jellyfish tentacle in the ear.'

As the team nervously laughed, I hoped my advice had served to break the tension but I also wanted to make an important point.

The idea of negative visualisation and preparing for the worst is a powerful practice used by ancient stoic philosophers. Known as *Premeditatio Malorum*, it literally translates as the 'pre-meditation of the evils and troubles that might lie ahead'.

This is why Seneca once wrote, 'What is quite unlooked for is more crushing in its effect, and unexpectedness adds to the weight of a disaster. This is a reason for ensuring that nothing ever takes us by surprise. We should project our thoughts ahead of us at every turn and have in mind every possible eventuality instead of only the usual course of events. Rehearse them in your mind: exile, torture, war, shipwreck. All the terms of our human lot should be before our eyes.'

This was something I practised before every sea swim.

No matter how short or seemingly simple, as an adventurer I would have rehearsed everything that could go wrong. Whether it was a visit from a curious bull shark in the Bahamas or a rogue tide that was sending me backwards faster than I could swim. I had thought about it all and now as a coach I encouraged my team to do the same.

By 4 p.m. the tide was high and the time for *Premeditatio Malorum* was over.

The sandy causeway connecting the island to the beach on the mainland known as Bigbury-on-Sea was now entirely underwater which meant the only way back to the mainland for the team was in a pair of goggles. Watching on from the support boat, my final words were 'to swim strong and stoic', no matter what the sea threw at them.

What followed was one of the hardest 1 km swims I've ever had to watch as a coach.

You see, unbeknown to me at the time, Tessa was suffering from food poisoning. But as one of the world's most experienced Olympians she was also aware how important it was to rehearse and replicate 'race conditions' during the *Peak Mesocycle* and so didn't want to miss the chance to complete her first sea swim.

So, she decided to keep it a secret from me and the team.

You cannot keep secrets from the sea. It's entirely unforgiving and if you have a weakness it will become highlighted, which is exactly what happened to Tessa. Only 400 metres into the swim, she was hit by a rogue wave as she turned her head to breathe. Choking and gasping for air, she swallowed so much saltwater that then mixed with the toxins from the food poisoning and began churning around in her stomach like a washing machine.

But a tormented tummy wasn't my only concern.

That's because on the starboard side of my boat, Arg was being pushed east by the tide, meaning unless he swam harder and faster he'd miss the beach and end up in Cornwall. Meanwhile, to the port side, Sair was engulfed in waves after swimming into choppy waters that flowed over a concealed sandbank.

Sensing the danger and unsure how to cope with the unique conditions of their new 'swimming pool' they stopped, began to panic and looked up at me for answers. But despite witnessing the fear in their eyes, my answer (and instruction) was very clear.

'Swim!' I shouted pointing in the direction of the beach.

Both looked startled at my abrupt reply and lack of empathy, but the truth is I wasn't being mean. Instead, while they floated there looking at me for answers, they were being pushed and pulled by the tides and waves and were completely at the mercy of the ocean. This is why I say, when it comes to sea swimming the answer is so often swim. The question is so often irrelevant.

- Bullied by the tide? Then swim yourself free of it.
- Feeling seasick with food poisoning? Then swim and it's over faster.

- Caught in choppy waters? Then swim yourself clear of the sandbank.
- Fatigued from swimming? Then swim some more and it's over quicker so you can rest.

Essentially, when quitting isn't an option, know that swimming is always your solution.

What I then witnessed over the next 30 minutes (and 1 km) was nothing short of heroic. Locked in their own personal battles with the sea, every one of the team refused to give up and made it back to shore with a profound understanding of *Premeditatio Malorum* having rehearsed and replicated 'race conditions'.

Watching as the team members hugged on the beach, in many ways their training had gone from a baptism to a graduation and an exorcism. Yes, this may sound dramatic, but one thing these swims had done was help to combat deep-routed 'demons' that had laid dormant in each team member for years. From Alex harbouring concerns about the functionality of his limbs that had been embedded in his psyche since childhood, to Arg's concern about his weight and level of fitness.

But perhaps the biggest psychological 'demon' that had been exorcised by over half the members of our team was the (incorrect) socially constructed stereotype that black people can't swim. According to a study published by Sport England, up to 95 per cent of black adults do not swim. Why? The truth is there are many reasons, but one (unfortunate) fact that cannot be ignored is the racist history that surrounds swimming, stemming back to segregation, when black people were not allowed to access swimming pools. This coupled with the false idea that black people are genetically predisposed to be bad at swimming and it's clear to see why swimming as a sport had become so divided.

But it didn't need to be and as the sun went down on Burgh Island, I gathered the team on the beach to tell them a story about one of the greatest and most inspiring swimmers I've ever trained with, a man called Jacques Sicot.

A local legend on the small island of Martinique, he stood 5 ft 9 in tall and despite being 70 years old had zero body fat and a complete disregard for the ageing process. Jacques Sicot was one of the Caribbean's greatest long-distance sea swimmers whose accolades include a circumnavigation swim around St Lucia. But what I loved most about Jacques was his love of the sea and how his love of swimming had been completely untainted by any negative stereotypes. Instead, each morning he would take his fishing boat out to sea, drop anchor, jump in and proceed to swim 10 km in crystal-clear blue water. With no history of racial segregation and no falsely circulated rumours concerning his genetic make-up, he continued to swim distances many people would consider impossible for a man of his age, race and ethnicity.

I then told the team our swim was now much more than a fundraising swim for an incredible cause. Instead, we were swimming as part of a media project broadcast to millions to try and 'turn the tide' on years of swimming segregation.

But my inspiring speech on the beach that day also came with a word of warning. Although I would never question the team's courage, I remained concerned about our speed (or our lack of it). Also, I knew the sea wouldn't care how noble our cause was or how much money we were trying to raise for charity. As far as Mother Nature and Poseidon were concerned, you either swim strong and at speed or you don't swim at all. Unfortunately, despite some truly courageous swims, I knew certain members of the team were not ready.

So, I then told the entire team that to even be allowed to attempt a crossing of the English Channel, every member of the relay must complete a two-hour qualifying swim in Loch Lomond in water temperatures of 15°C (60°F) or less and then record and register that swim with the Channel Swimming Association.

Sensing we were now at the business end of our macrocycle (year's training) we then headed north to Scotland. Once there, every member of the team would have to honestly ask themselves if they were truly ready.

THE POWER OF THE 1 PER CENT

SUMMER 2019, LOCH LOMOND, SCOTLAND

It was 18 August 2019 and we had arrived in Scotland. Looking out across the mass expanse of water, you couldn't help but feel small and humbled by the beauty of the Highlands as the mountains tower overhead and plunge into the valley below that is home to Loch Lomond. At 36.4 km (22.6 miles) long and up to 8 km (4.97 miles) wide, it's considered the largest lake in Great Britain by surface area and attracts over 4 million visitors a year who flock to walk the adventure trails, sample the local cuisine and sail the loch.

But today, myself and the team had no time for tourism. Instead, ice cream and sightseeing would have to wait since we had a two-hour English Channel qualification swim to conquer, and the arrival of our support boats signalled that preparation was about to begin.

Walking down to the water's edge I didn't say a word, mainly because I didn't have to. After weeks of coaching, I had seen a group of individuals evolve into a team of genuine sea swimmers. As a result, they knew exactly how to prep and plan before every swim and didn't need me to hold their hand any more. Like a proud parent, I just watched on.

Alex sat on the floor and began to make the necessary adjustments to his prosthetic swimming leg. Now so comfortable and confident in the water, he assembled it like a special forces sniper would assemble a gun. Equally, Rachel was now able to tie her long, braided hair into a bun and wrap it in a swimming cap with military precision.

But perhaps my favourite moment that day when watching on as a coach was when the entire team banded together to apply lubricating Vaseline to Arg's arms and legs. Yes, that sounds odd I know. Yes, it might seem strange to many, but the reason I was so proud of Arg's lubricated armpits and groin was because they were almost symbolic of the team's transition to become fully-sledged sea swimmers. Forgoing the social norms of society, athletes of this sport are a different breed. We casually lube each other up like it's normal, defecate while swimming without breaking stroke and during really cold swims will even urinate on our own hands to warm them up.

This is all because to us, it's not strange; to us it's *The Power of the 1 per cent* when sea swimming. Inspired by the great Sir Clive Woodward who coached the England rugby team to World Cup victory in 2003, it's this idea that so often coaches and athletes look to make big, grand changes to their training to improve performance whereas, in reality, making small 1 per cent improvements across many areas can result in a huge cumulative increase in overall performance.

A pioneer of this philosophy, Woodward's attention to detail, preparation and culture of professionalism was legendary. Perhaps the best example of this is when he recruited a 'vision awareness coach' for every single player in his team. Yes, that's right, a coach recruited to specifically train the eyeballs of his players. Her name was Dr Sherylle Calder, a guru in vision awareness who said, 'The concept is to get the eye to pick up the ball early and to judge early . . . it's not just the ability to be physically quicker, but seeing the play early and getting to the right place at the right time.' She added, 'I see my job with England as adding that little edge. If you improve a player by 1 per cent, you make him better than he was and one decision wins a World Cup.'

In short, they searched for marginal improvements anywhere and everywhere. Which is why although incremental gains in the form of correctly fitted prosthetic legs and suitably lubricated armpits might seem trivial, when out at sea among tides, currents, waves and weather they can have a profound impact on overall performance.

But even when fully prepared with (seemingly) no stone left unturned, certain members of the team were about to discover things can still go very wrong during a long swim and when they do, you have to honestly ask yourself if you're ready.

ARE YOU READY FOR THIS?

The time was 1 p.m. and the qualification swim was about to start. Since it was summertime in Scotland, the water was 60°F (15.5°C) which wasn't freezing but certainly wasn't tropical either. This is why I warned every member of the team that they must keep a good pace throughout the two hours in order to cover a good distance, but equally to generate heat and ward off hypothermia.

'How fast do I need to go?' Linford asked while reminding me his Jamaican genetics were not built to be swimming in cold Scottish lochs.

'Fast enough so you can always feel your hands and feet ideally,' I replied.

He nodded but looked concerned as he tightened the zip on his wetsuit, anticipating the next two hours would be the coldest of his life. As he did, the entire team began checking goggles, hats and ear plugs as they collectively practised *Premeditatio Malorum* knowing this swim would be taking them into completely uncharted waters.

But it wasn't just the team that were pre-meditating the evils that might lie ahead; I too was preparing myself to console those who wouldn't make it. Of course, I wanted to remain optimistic and as a friend and coach I wanted to see everyone make the final relay team. But as a sports scientist studying the science and psychology of adventure I also knew this wouldn't be the case.

Why was I so sure? Every member of the team had trained so hard, sacrificed so much and never missed a single training session, so surely that would mean everyone deserved to qualify, join the final team and stand on the white cliffs of Dover, right? Well, unfortunately no. Not when you consider the findings of the HERITAGE Family Study.[275]

In this large-scale study conducted from 1992 to 2004, sports scientists took 120 separate publications and investigated the role of genotype – the genetic make-up of an individual – in mediating exercise response to endurance training. They decided to measure people's change in maximal oxygen uptake. This is their lung capacity, VO2 max, and an increase in this is a good indication of someone improving their cardiovascular fitness.

Amazingly, what they found was the average increase in VO2 max was 19 per cent. However, scientists noted that 5 per cent of participants had little or no change in VO2 max and 5 per cent had an increase of 40 to 50 per cent and more, despite each person being subjected to the same training programme and stimulus. Basically, there was huge inter-individual variability and if represented in a graph, it would be difficult to discern a pattern.

Scientists concluded, 'Previously it was assumed that these variations result from differing degrees of compliance with the training program, i.e., good compliers have the highest percentage of improvement and poor compliers show little or no improvement. However, it is now clear that even when there is full compliance with the program, substantial variations occur in the percentage improvements in VO2 max values of different people.'

Importantly, strength training produces the exact same inter-individual variability.

This is based on research published in the *Journal of Medicine and Science in Sport* where scientists studied the strength training adaptations of 585 young men and women who followed a 12-week training plan. They discovered the average strength gain was 54 per cent.[276]

This sounds great, right? Well, yes, but the improvements ranged from 0 and 250 per cent.

The same was found in a study of 23 elite rugby players too.[277] Researchers wanted to test the hormonal response to four different weight-training protocols. So, they examined testosterone (one of our muscle-building hormones) and cortisol (our 'stress hormone') in players before, immediately after and 30 minutes later once they'd completed the following regimes (each one consisting of four exercises: bench press, leg press, seated row and squats):

- FOUR sets of 10 repetitions at 70 per cent of 1RM with 2 minutes' rest between sets.
- THREE sets of five reps at 85 per cent 1RM with 3 minutes' rest.
- FIVE sets of 15 reps at 55 per cent 1RM with 1 minute's rest.
- THREE sets of five reps at 40 per cent 1RM with 3 minutes' rest.

The result? Again, massive inter-individual variation among each athlete as researchers concluded, despite being from the same team, 'Individual athletes differed in their hormonal response to each of the protocols.'

All of this explains why one hour into the swim, Tessa and Diane bowed out.

Two members of the team who had trained so hard, had always given 100 per cent and never missed a single training session, but despite this weren't able to reach the two-hour qualifying standard based on what we learnt from the HERITAGE Family study.

Hugging them aboard the boat, I could see they were upset.

'We didn't qualify?' Tessa replied confused, as if she was stating the obvious.

'Yes, maybe,' I confessed. 'But 12 weeks ago, you couldn't swim the length of a swimming pool. Today you both swam for an entire hour in one of Scotland's most iconic lochs and, in the process, have likely inspired thousands of young black girls to begin swimming.'

A small smile then appeared across their faces.

'What you've done is nothing short of heroic and should be cele-brated,' I continued. 'Because whether you qualified or not, you have achieved eudaimonia through askēsis. What's more, at 60 and 64 years old you have both added another amazing adventure onto a highly decorated athletic and media career.'

Their smiles then began to broaden.

Tessa was one of Britain's greatest Olympians and Diane was one of Britain's longest-serving and beloved TV presenters, therefore they both knew it was right for them (and the team) that their adventures ended among the green Highlands and crystal-clear waters of Loch Lomond.

Delivering them back to shore with a final hug, my attention then turned back to the remaining members of the team who were now just 50 minutes away from completing their qualifying swim. Desperate to ensure no-one else dropped out, I could see fatigue (and the cold) was creeping in as their swimming strokes began to break down.

'Keep swimming!' I shouted.

'Do not touch the boat under any circumstances,' I then said, reminding them this would result in an immediate disqualification.

For the next 10 minutes, I continued yelling instructions that echoed throughout the loch and with 40 minutes remaining I even began to allow myself to dream of the finish line, but this was a mistake. As I did, disaster struck in the form of Alex's troubled bowels.

'What's wrong?' I asked as he came to an abrupt stop.

'It's my stomach,' he said. 'I think I've got food poisoning from a questionable burger I had.'

'Ok, ok, don't panic,' I replied as I assessed our options.

Looking around, the harsh reality is there were none. If he got out or touched the boat he would be disqualified, and if he stopped swimming he'd start getting cold fast could develop hypothermia. I decided that our only option was not a pleasant one.

'Listen, if you have to take a shit in your wetsuit, just do it. But whatever you do, do not stop swimming and do not touch this boat.'

'But I can't take a shit here,' he insisted.

Understanding it's not the solution he hoped for, I assured him that it was fine.

'Don't worry, we can deal with the consequences after and I'll hose you down,' I said.

'No, you don't understand,' Alex paused while trying to decide how best to tell me his predicament.

'My grandad's ashes were scattered here . . . I can't shit on my grandad.'

I stood there stunned into silence. In all of my years of coaching and swimming, this was a problem I'd never come across before.

'Ok, you're just going to have to swim, clench your butt cheeks and think of your grandad,' I said.

Alex nodded. He knew what he had to do.

For the next 40 minutes, I then witnessed a truly heroic swim. Powering through the loch, lap after lap, I have absolutely no doubt Alex's grandad was watching on with pride as his grandson overcame food poisoning, any perceived disability and the past trauma of childhood swimming lessons gone wrong. Fuelled by a resolute refusal to quit, for the remaining minutes neither his tightly clenched butt cheeks or swim stroke faltered as his wetsuit remained unsoiled.

Then, just like that, the alarm on my stopwatch signalled it was over.

Cheers erupted from across the loch. We started this entire adventure with 11 individual swimmers who could barely swim a lap of a pool, but after 12 weeks of training we now had a united team of eight who would travel to Dover to attempt to cross the English Channel.

With all the hard work done, the team now had to learn to taper their training as we would be leaving for Dover in 10 days' time and attempting to swim 21 miles (34 km) to Calais, following in the footsteps of the great Captain Matthew Webb.

PLAN TO PEAK

SUMMER 2019, (ALL OVER) ENGLAND

We were 10 days away from our relay swim across the English Channel. Every member of the team had returned home, which meant I spent this entire time travelling the length and breadth of England ensuring everyone (including myself, but still undercover) was lowering the volume of their training, while keeping intensity high and drilling *Specific Physical Preparedness*. Why? Because the objective of any training programme is to peak for a specific adventure/competition. It's essentially the final piece of the puzzle that is your macrocycle (year's training plan), where you manipulate training variables in order to achieve a temporary state where physical and psychological elements are maximised and levels of technical and tactical preparation are optimal.

Put simply, it's the final few weeks of your *Peak Mesocycle* that ensure you arrive on the start line, at the base of your mountain or (in our case) by the water's edge looking out to sea, fully rested, fully prepared and 'ready for war'. Too often, people neglect this and wonder why they bomb on the day of competition or during an expedition.

So how do we 'peak'?

Different athletes and adventurers will use different methods to peak, but the basic theory is always the same. The underlying component of the ability to peak is one's 'preparedness', which is the ability of the body to actually exert itself maximally. Preparedness can be further broken down into the sum of 'fitness' (how well developed your ability to move your body actually is, in this case your strength) and 'fatigue' (the depletion of energy substrates

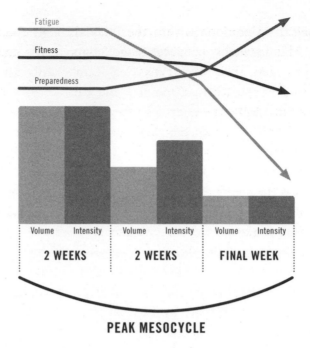

PEAK MESOCYCLE

and damage to the muscles, hormonal axes and nervous system that impede fitness expression). Represented in a graph, if an athlete's *Peak Mesocycle* was five weeks long, it could (in theory) look like the figure above.

You'll notice from the graph that the volume of training is initially reduced more than the intensity of training. The reason for this is that research shows that volume (*not* intensity) is the primary contributor to fatigue. As a result, the exact training programme was a stripped-back, tapered-down version of the *Build Mesocycle* where:

- The number of strength sessions per week are reduced.
- Sets and repetitions within those sessions are reduced.
- Total mileage of swimming per week is tapered down.

This is all because during the *Build Mesocycle* (as the intensity was increased and volume was kept high) the goal was to stimulate physiological adaptations within the body through the stress of training. This inevitably produces some fatigue as the muscles run low on glycogen, their fibre types may temporarily alter to the weaker kind (Type IIb to Type IIa) and they accumulate micro tears. Basically, while the body is getting stronger, faster and fitter, your actual ability to express these new-found physical capabilities can be hidden by the fatigue that this very training serves to generate.

Therefore, the goal to 'peaking' is to *maintain* fitness with none of the fatigue, which myself and the team were going to achieve with the following workout.

PEAK TRAINING PLAN (SUMMER): MICROCYCLE (WEEK'S PLAN)
HOW TO PEAK: THE FORMAT

The microcycle contains SEVEN sessions per week which consists of:

- TWO strength (and speed) sessions primarily for the maintenance of fitness.
- TWO slow and long (5 km) open-water swims (ideally at sea) operating in Zone 2 to maintain the solid aerobic base ('gas tank'), but the main focus is on perfecting Specific Physical Preparedness (to ensure levels of technical and tactical preparation are optimal).
- THREE high-intensity interval sessions operating in Zones 4 and 5 to maintain anaerobic fitness (add some 'jet engine afterburners' to the already sizeable 'gas tank').

With all of this represented in a table, a week's training looks like this:

	Monday	Tuesday	Wednesday	Thursday	Friday	Saturday	Sunday
MORNING	Swim Interval Training	Swim 5km Open Water	Swim Interval Training	Swim 5km Open Water	Swim Interval Training	REST	REST
PURPOSE	Anaerobic Fitness (Zones 4 & 5)	Aerobic Fitness (Zone 2)	Anaerobic Fitness (Zones 4 & 5)	Aerobic Fitness (Zone 2)	Anaerobic Fitness (Zones 4 & 5)		
AFTERNOON	Upper Body		Lower-Body Routine				
PURPOSE	Supplementary Strength and Speed Training		Supplementary Strength and Speed Training				

5-DAY BASE PROGRAMME

AEROBIC FITNESS: 5 KM SWIM (ZONE 2)

Exercises	Time	Distance	Intensity
Swim	60+ minutes	5 km	Zone 2 60–70 per cent of your maximum heart rate

Coaching Cues

These sessions operate in Zone 2 to maintain a solid aerobic base and 'gas tank' (your heart, lungs and cardiorespiratory system) while also maintaining Specific Physical Preparedness and swimming technique focusing on body position, breathing, arm stroke and leg kick.

ANAEROBIC FITNESS: HIGH-INTENSITY INTERVALS (ZONES 4 AND 5)

Exercises	Intervals	Time	Distance	Intensity
WARM-UP	1 km	15–20 minutes	1 km	Zone 2 60–70 per cent of your maximum heart rate

Coaching Cues

The purpose of the warm-up is to acclimatise to the cold water (if being performed in a lake or the sea) and to help prepare the body for the session ahead by raising your body temperature and increasing blood flow to your muscles.

Exercises	Intervals	Time	Distance	Intensity
TECHNIQUE	10 x 200 m	30–40 minutes	2 km	Zone 3 70–80 per cent of your maximum heart rate

Coaching Cues

The primary goal here to maintain Specific Physical Preparedness by drilling an efficient technique at a faster pace. Focusing specifically on body position, breathing, arm stroke and leg kick.

Exercises	Intervals	Time	Distance	Intensity
MAIN SET	10 x 200 m	30 minutes	2 km	Zones 4 and 5 80–100 per cent of your maximum heart rate

Coaching Cues

This is the most important part of the entire session. This is where oxygen use increases, heart rate elevates, fuel is burnt, chemicals build up which contribute to exhaustion, water is lost, heat accumulates, muscles fatigue and the molecular energy of the muscles (adenosine triphosphate) runs low. But finishing this will ensure you maintain your anaerobic fitness ('jet engine afterburners') and maintain the buffering capacity of your muscles to cope with fatigue.

Exercises	Intervals	Time	Distance	Intensity
COOL-DOWN	500 m	10 minutes	500 m	Zones 1 and 2 50–70 per cent of your maximum heart rate

Coaching Cues

The goal of a cool-down is to reduce heart and breathing rates, gradually cool body temperature, return muscles to their optimal length–tension relationships and restore physiologic systems close to baseline as you prepare to 'switch on' the parasympathetic nervous system and begin the recovery process.

MONDAY: UPPER BODY

SUPPLEMENTARY STRENGTH AND SPEED TRAINING

Exercises	Repetitions	Sets	Rest	Physiological Adaptation
Passive Hang (Brachiating) (p 301)	60 seconds	3	90 seconds	Strength Rehab/ Prehab
Scapula Pull-Ups (p 302)	10	3	90 seconds	Strength Rehab/ Prehab
Overhead Medicine Ball Slams (p 303)	4–6	3	90 seconds	Speed-Strength Training Zone
Overhand (Pronated) Weighted Pull-Ups (p 303)	8–10	3	90 seconds	Strength-Speed Training Zone
Band-Resisted Single Arm Rows (p 309)	4–6	3	90 seconds	Peak Power Training
Scapula Push-Ups (p 319)	10	3	90 seconds	Strength Rehab/ Prehab
Plyometric Push-Ups (p 321)	5	3	90 seconds	Speed-Strength Training Zone
Band-Resisted Push-Ups (p 321)	8–10	3	90 seconds	Strength Training Zone
Band-Resisted Tricep Push-Downs (p 325)	12	3	60 seconds	Peak Power Training Zone

WEDNESDAY: LOWER BODY ROUTINE

SUPPLEMENTARY STRENGTH AND SPEED TRAINING

Exercises	Repetitions	Sets	Rest	Physiological Adaptation
Box Jumps (p 315)	5–7	3	120 seconds	Speed-Strength Training Zone
Single-Arm Dumbbell Side Lunge and Touch (p 316)	10 (each side)	3	90 seconds	Stability Strength, Posture and Body Position
Battle Rope Wrestler Throws (p 317)	8 (each side)	3	90 seconds	Speed-Strength Training Zone
Stability Ball Log Roll (p 317)	60 seconds	3	90 seconds	Stability Strength, Posture and Body Position
Pallof Hold and Press (p 318)	60 seconds	3	90 seconds	Stability Strength, Posture and Body Position

PREPARE FOR WAR, BUT PRAY FOR PEACE

AUGUST 2019, DOVER, ENGLAND

It was 29 August 2019 and we had arrived in Dover, England. Located on Kent's south coast, this small coastal town is home to one of the busiest ferry ports in the world. Being the closest point to continental Europe, an estimated 11.7 million passengers, 2.6 million lorries, 2.2 million cars and 80,000 coaches pass through this port each year. But today, we hoped to add 'relay team' to that list and in the process:

- Raise money for cancer research.
- 'Turn the tide' on negative stereotypes surrounding swimming.
- Change people's preconceived ideas about an ideal body shape/ style for swimming.
- See each team member achieve a profound sense of eudaimonia.

By 10 a.m. we had gathered at the small cottage we'd rented. Situated on the beachfront, this would serve as our headquarters as we sat, ate and waited to see when (and if) we'd be allowed to start our Channel crossing. When attempting to cross the Channel, it's not you who dictates the start time. No, it's Mother Nature and Poseidon, so we had to wait for our boat's pilot (registered with the Channel Swimming Association) to inform us if we had a weather window to attempt the 21 mile (34 km) swim. Now this weather window could be midday or midnight. But I knew when the tide, weather and waves all changed in our favour, we needed to be waving goodbye to the white cliffs of Dover and heading to Calais, France.

Back at the cottage I commandeered a quiet corner, opened my laptop and then began religiously monitoring tidal charts and weather reports. Keeping one eye on the charts and another on the team, I could see they were getting collectively more nervous, anxious and irritable with every hour that passed. It was like watching a group of caged animals who each possessed a different coping strategy unique to them.

Linford, for example, remained quiet and stoic. In fact, he was so relaxed he'd often drift in and out of sleep napping on the sofa. Meanwhile, Arg had decided to pass the time by arranging a local tanning salon to visit the cottage to administer a spray tan. All the while, Wes was hard at work on his phone arranging the after-party in London once we returned from Calais.

I'll be honest, I wasn't immune to the tension either. Now so invested in the team's success, I did my best to keep my emotions 'bottled up' as the goggles and swim hat in my bag remained a secret that I hoped I'd never have to use.

But at midday lunch was served, with a side helping of hope.

As rice, chicken and dumplings were dished out, I got a phone call from our captain who informed me we had a weather window of 5 p.m. that night. Turning to the team, I then told them this was very likely to be our last supper on English soil before the swim. After a few moments' silence, (inevitably) a barrage of questions were thrown my way.

'What time will we be back?' Wes asked.

'Why?' I replied confused.

'Because I need to know for the after-party,' he said, as if it was obvious.

I smiled, not wanting to dampen his confidence. But I told him that back in 1875 when Captain Matthew Webb dived off the pier in Dover, he probably wasn't thinking about the guest list to his after-party, so I advised Wes to focus on the swim and not the celebration.

'I've a question,' Arg said looking troubled.

Praying it wasn't about a party and hoping it was swim related, I then encouraged him to voice his concern to the group in case it was a question that was on everyone's minds.

'Will my spray tan be dry by then?'

I shouldn't have laughed, but I couldn't help it.

'Arg, the honest answer is I don't know,' I said, now trying to bring some much-needed professionalism back to the dinner table. 'I'm a swim coach, not a tanning expert. I don't care whether you're a shade of pink, brown or a rich mahogany, at 5 p.m. I want you prepped and ready.'

SETTING SAIL

It was 4 p.m. and our final preparations had begun. Shuttling kit, food and other provisions from the car park to the harbour, thankfully talk of after-parties had ceased for the time being and spray tans had also dried, so Arg (now an impressive shade of mocha) could now focus on the task at hand.

But that evening we weren't the only ones preparing for our crossing. Looking across the harbour, I noticed two other boats were being stocked and prepped, clearly trying to capitalise on the weather window just like us. Wanting to offer some support, I took a moment to walk over and wish them luck, since I've always felt a sense of solidarity among sea swimmers that bonds complete strangers, no matter what age, shape, size or nationality.

But aboard the boats I found something I wasn't expecting . . . 12 pupils from Taunton Preparatory School in Somerset. All were wearing matching uniforms, most of them were tiny and the youngest was a shy, softly spoken 12-year-old girl who was carb-loading on a bag of jelly babies. Wired on sugar, she then told me their swim was to raise money for the Neonatal Unit at Musgrove Park Hospital (where many of them were born) which was as inspiring as it was incredibly sweet. Sharing a bag of toffee while exchanging sea swimming stories, I wished them luck and said I hoped to see them in Calais.

By 4.45 p.m. I was back on our boat and we were ready to leave.

Pulling out of the marina we headed to a point on the coast called Shakespeare Cliff. A small, short stretch of shingle beach to the west of Dover Harbour, this is where most Channel swims begin as the cliff offers some shelter from the northerly wind and drops you straight into favourable tides, which (in theory) all makes for a smooth start.

Not just a smooth start either, but a beautiful one.

That afternoon we were gifted with the most incredible view from the boat's deck. With the sun getting lower in the sky, it illuminated one of our country's most famous landmarks: the White Cliffs of Dover. Officially declared an icon of Britain, the cliffs themselves are made of a very pure form of limestone and tower 106 metres (348 ft) above the sea. Owing their striking appearance to the composition of chalk accentuated by streaks of black flint, the cliffs are recognised throughout the world and have been witness to some of the most dramatic moments in English history, from the arrival of the Romans to the return of the British forces from Dunkirk during World War II. In my opinion, the English Channel is one of the greatest 'swimming pools' on planet earth purely based on its history and heritage.

But we hadn't come here for sightseeing. We had a Channel to swim, money to raise and people (of all ages and ethnicities) to inspire, which is why moments later we were watching Wes as he stepped foot on the beach to start our aquatic adventure.

'Are you ready?' I shouted from the boat.

Wes put on his goggles, tightened his hat and signalled he was.

My heart was beating out of my chest. I've never been so nervous before a swim but continued to compose myself for the good of the team. Noting the exact start time on my watch with military precision so I could manage the one-hour intervals each team member must swim, I then instructed Wes to get into the water and begin our campaign to Calais.

Starting strong, as predicted he was shielded from the wind by Shakespeare Cliff and dived straight into a favourable tide. Watching on from the boat, we then saw others begin their swim from the beach too, as three other teams began their Channel attempts, each trying to take advantage of the few remaining weather windows left of the English summer.

Among them were the kids of Taunton School. Taking off like a shot, their lead swimmer ploughed through the water like a missile, overtaking Wes at a rate of knots. All I could do was wave and wish them luck as they disappeared over the horizon still fuelled on jelly babies and toffee.

I won't lie, I was so happy for them . . . but now worried for us.

I had always been so concerned about the team's speed, but now those fears were turning into reality as I watched Wes (one of our strongest swimmers) get rapidly overtaken by a primary school relay team. An hour passed and Wes put in a solid performance and then handed over to Greg. Climbing onto the boat, Wes turned to me.

'How was that?' he asked, eager to know of our progress.

'Really good,' I replied.

'Did you see that beast overtake me?' he continued.

I nodded, but didn't say a word. I didn't want him to know the 'beast' he was referring to was likely a 12-year-old boy or girl from Somerset, since I didn't know how that news would be handled by the group so early into our swim. Instead, I instructed him to get warm and eat. We had eight team members in total, swimming in hour-long intervals, which meant Wes would be back in the water in seven hours' time so needed to remain focused.

I then politely excused myself and headed to the galley of the boat to run the numbers on the swimming statistics of our first swim. As I thought, it wasn't good. Based on our current speeds, we were going to be out here for more than 24 hours.

This was no longer a swim, it was going to be a war of attrition.

THE MATHS AND MAPS

It was around 7.45 p.m. and progress was slow, but steady. I had been bouncing about the boat attending to my various coaching duties as I supervised those in the water from the deck and forecasted our progress from the galley. But with each hour that passed, I was becoming more and more nervous that Calais (and our hopes of crossing the Channel) was slipping through our fingers.

So far, we had covered only 4.1 miles (6.6 km) in almost three hours. Therefore, based on our average speed, it would take us over 28 hours to swim the total 21 miles (34 km) to Calais. But what's worse is that didn't account for the added distance travelled caused by the tides and the S-shaped course we'd be forced to swim (that I'd previously warned the team about way back in Windermere during interval training). Also, with slower members of the team still yet to swim, it meant our average speed would drop further and that S-shape would become more pronounced, adding more miles to the journey, as we would get pushed and pulled by the tide.

Perhaps the best example of this was the contrasting speed and total distances covered by two very different (but equally heroic) swims: Roger Allsopp and Trent Grimsey.

On 31 August 2011, Roger Allsopp became the oldest person to swim the Channel (at the time), completing his crossing in 17 hours and 51 minutes and 19 seconds at 70 years of age. Raising money for

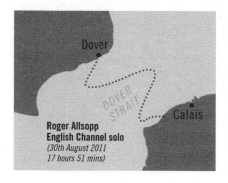

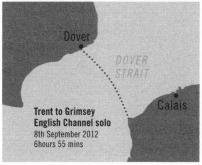

breast cancer research, it was a remarkable achievement, but when you compare his S-shaped route to the current world record, it's clear to see how swimming at speed is far more efficient.

That's because in comparison, on 8 September 2012, Australian-born Trent Grimsey ploughed through the water like a speedboat and reached Calais in a time of 6 hours and 55 minutes, shaving a full 2 minutes off the previous record held by Bulgarian Petar Stoychev. As he was travelling so fast, the map plotting his route shows no S-shape, just a slight bend, showing he was virtually unaffected by the tides.

But right now, we were travelling at 1.37 mph (2.2 km/h) and it was very likely our route would be even more divergent than Roger Allsopp's. With a pencil, I carefully drew our route on the map and realised we needed a solution. Visiting the galley, Caroline (executive producer) saw the map and immediately realised this too.

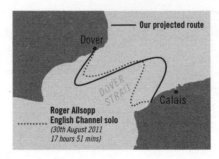

'Do you have your kit?' she asked.

I reluctantly nodded.

'I do, but this is still their adventure. I'll only jump in if I absolutely have to. Otherwise I'll be robbing them of their chance to achieve eudaimonia if I just swim a big "chunk" of it.'

She nodded and understood.

Every member of the team had trained so hard and each of them deserved to stand on the coast of Calais for the hours and miles they'd sacrificed for this swim.

'So, what's your plan?' she asked.

Pausing for a moment I realised we needed some swims of heroic proportions to propel us closer to France . . . and we needed them now. Thankfully, as the sun began to set in the sky, heroes emerged from within our ranks.

NOT ALL HEROES WEAR CAPES, SOME WEAR GOGGLES

It was 7.55 p.m. and we were prepping for the relay's next changeover. This was becoming a tad trickier as the sun began to set at sea and Mother Nature prepared to 'turn the lights off'. Once she did, we'd be relying on head torches, lights mounted on the side of the boat and the team's innate sense of direction when swimming through the night. What this meant was we didn't just need a strong swim, we needed a superhuman swim.

Thankfully, I knew just the man.

Granted, he wasn't your conventional superhero type. He didn't have a cape and there were no comic books written in his honour. Instead, he came equipped with tight, bright yellow swimming trunks, a pair of goggles and the greatest spray tan in the history of sea swimming. Yes, my secret weapon was James (Arg) Argent.

'Big man, we need a huge swim from you,' I said, looking him dead in the eyes.

'How big?' he asked.

'Gigantic,' I replied sternly. 'I don't want to panic you, but even at this early stage our Channel hopes may be resting on those big shoulders of yours. So, for one hour, I need you to swim strong and at speed. I need you take a massive "bite" out of the distance covered and get us closer to Calais. Ok?'

He nodded and then (knowing his swim would have a profound impact on our Channel hopes) began to adjust his hat, tighten his goggles and lubricate his armpits.

By 7.59 p.m. he was poised on the side of the boat, ready to jump in. Keeping to a tight schedule, I began the countdown.

'Three, two, one . . . GO! GO! GO!' I shouted.

My voice echoed across the ocean and as instructed Arg took off like a navy missile. Ploughing through the water with big, powerful strokes, after months of training both his 'gas tank' (aerobic energy system) and 'jet engine afterburners' (anaerobic energy system) were working beautifully and I couldn't have been prouder.

There was just one issue though . . . he was going the wrong way.

Entirely amped up on adrenaline, yet confused by the fading light, my secret weapon had completely misfired and was swimming back to Dover. Rushing to the helm of the boat, I began shouting, desperate to turn him around.

'ARG! ARG! YOU'RE GOING THE WRONG WAY!'

Eventually, he stopped and lifted his head from the water.

'What?' he asked confused.

'France is THAT way,' I said pointing in the other direction.

'Oh, ok, thank you,' he replied, before turning a full 180 degrees and continuing with his incredible speed, just now in the right direction.

Inspired by Arg's swim, other team members followed and through the night I recorded more personal bests and top speeds for everyone. As a coach, I couldn't have been prouder, but somewhere between midnight and sunrise I began to sense trouble was on the horizon and I started to wonder if the team's best would be enough.

GO DOWN 'SWIMMING'?

The time was 3.55 p.m. and we were prepping for another changeover. Only this time our transition wouldn't be as smooth. That's because we had covered 13 miles (21 km) in 11 hours and now found ourselves almost directly in the middle of the English Channel. As a result, the coastline no longer sheltered us from the wind which meant we had no option but to go over, through or under the waves that were now plaguing our swim.

To make matters worse the tide had now changed and was beginning to take us way off course, and if we continued on our current route, we'd miss Calais and end up in Dunkirk or even worse Belgium. Hoping and praying the turbulent waters would pass, I turned to the team in need of yet another hero, since the reality was I didn't just need them to swim, I needed them to survive and hold our position. Moments later, as if on cue one appeared on deck with goggles in one hand and a prosthetic leg in the other.

'This is going to hurt, isn't it?' Alex asked.

'Yes,' I replied unable to lie, but also keen to practise *Premeditatio Malorum*.

'This won't just be a swim, it will be a fight,' I said.

Alex nodded, fully accepted his fate and without a moment's hesitation jumped off the side of the boat to take one for the team. Immediately engulfed by the water, he got slapped across the face with a huge wave that knocked his goggles clean off his face.

Taking it like a champ, he had a granite chin that any heavyweight boxer would love to possess. Signalling he was okay, he then proceeded to swim backstroke (his preferred technique) towards France like a Viking warship, breaking the waves with his head and shoulders with an unrelenting stroke which you could set your watch to.

An hour later, Alex had finished his relay leg. Clambering onto the boat bruised and battered, he and the team had been quite literally fighting from dusk till dawn to maintain our course. But come 7 a.m. things went from bad to worse, because as the sun began to rise, so did the wind and waves.

Looking at the map, I urged the team to go on fighting.

We had swum 16 miles (26 km) in total, but looking at the horizon our progress and the heroics of the night swims were even more apparent as the sun served to reveal the finish line to us in the form of Cap Gris Nez. In fact, we were so close that with every swim relay you could see a greater level of detail among the buildings and beaches and if you focused really hard, you could even see larger vehicles driving down the coast.

Swim after swim, the team came nearer and nearer to the beach.

But Mother Nature had other ideas and by 10.14 a.m., with Rachel now in the water, we had reached a form of 'swimming stalemate'. The tide had turned and was now pushing us back towards Dover, and with a swimming speed of 2–3 km/h it meant Rachel couldn't make any progress and all she could do was hold our position.

Watching on from the boat, I knew she was utterly fearless and possessed a resolute refusal to quit. But I also knew as the waves and swell of the sea increased, we would have trouble seeing her which meant difficult conditions could very quickly turn to outright dangerous ones.

TO SWIM OR NOT TO SWIM?

The time was 10.31 a.m. and the team had swum 18 miles (29 km) in total. Rachel was now really struggling to hold her position and we'd just received news over the radio that a storm was coming in from the south. With years of sea swimming experience in English waters, I knew this meant this particular swim was slipping through our fingers as we were beginning to lose the 'war to the shore'. Deciding I was more help to Rachel (and the team) in the water, I ripped open my bag and began searching for goggles.

'I'm getting in,' I said to Caroline.

'To swim it?' she asked.

'No, just to support her,' I replied.

I still desperately wanted the team to succeed without any intervention from me or anyone else. But I needed to get in the water to assist a teammate. Reaching Rachel, I could see she was distressed and disorientated as the waves were now so big she couldn't see the boat or the coastline so had no idea in which direction to swim.

'Follow me!' I shouted, while being careful not to touch her and risk disqualification.

With her sense of direction restored, she nodded and then continued the swim and struggle towards France. Battling fatigue and sleep deprivation, the waves continued to crash into her shoulders testing both her tendons and willpower.

Fifteen minutes passed and as I swam by her side I couldn't have been any prouder as a coach. The ocean had been trying to break the collective resolve of the team for hours now, yet swim after swim, each member of the team refused to give up for their peers.

I can only describe what I saw as pure heroism.

Which is what made accepting the data on my GPS watch even harder. With a heavy heart, I knew statistics didn't lie and based on the readings from my watch it was clear that Rachel was now going backwards. And the team would continue to do so, once the storm arrived from the south, basically pushing us back to Dover.

The captain, crew and Caroline knew this too.

'Ross!' Caroline shouted from the boat. 'I'm so sorry, but for safety reasons we're going to have to cancel the swim.'

At first, I didn't reply.

This was partly because I refused to accept defeat, but also because I wanted to stall in order to come up with a solution. Floating in the sea, I looked at the coastline ahead and quickly ran the numbers in my head. Knowing we had 5 km (3.1 miles) left, it seemed so close. Quite literally within touching distance. I could sprint to the end and be done in less than an hour.

But as I looked at the boat, I realised that although I could . . . I wasn't sure that I should.

Based on everything that I had learned about the science and psychology of adventure, it was clear that if I was to swim the remaining part of the relay I would be robbing the team of their chance to achieve eudaimonia. Yes, we might stand in Calais and return to an after-party (arranged by Wes), but this would be happiness without fulfilment and as a coach I couldn't do that to the team.

Yes, it was not a fairy-tale ending . . . but it was the right ending.

As expected, it was a slow and sombre boat journey back to Dover. Barely a word was spoken. After weeks, months and miles of training, it makes defeat in sea swimming even harder to accept. But the reality was, although their feet never touched French soil, this swim was a success based on every other metric. This is because they had:

- Raised thousands of pounds for cancer research.
- Combated negative stereotypes and inspired millions to swim.
- Swum 18 miles (29 km) *in* the English Channel (albeit not entirely *across* it).
- Achieved a profound sense of individual eudaimonia (through askēsis).

What's more, unbeknown to them at the time, they'd also truly inspired *me*.

They had set out on a personal journey of self-improvement, self-discipline and self-discovery, but in the process had collectively contributed to a cause far bigger than themselves.

It was essentially an adventure for a higher purpose.

Wanting to follow in their footsteps, I now knew that if I was to train for another athletic adventure of my own, it would have to be for a higher purpose too. Which is why after studying *How to Adventure*, the final things you must consider are *When to Adventure* and *Where to Adventure.*

PART 3 |
WHEN TO ADVENTURE

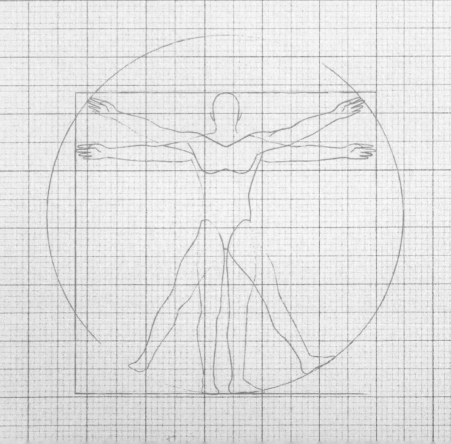

With coaching duties over, I refocused on my own training. Now adamant that I wanted to put my goggles and trunks on for a swim of significance, I began researching dates and locations and a new mesocycle so I could plot and plan my training in its entirety.

However, there was a problem in 2020 and it came in the form of COVID-19 which meant international travel and adventure was impossible to certain parts of the world. What's worse, my dad was continuing to battle cancer, which meant being in England with him and the family was more important right now.

So, all things considered (for me and many), 2020 was *not* the year to adventure.

How did I structure my training with no swim, date or location? Well, I decided there was no need for a *Recovery Mesocycle* (since I didn't actually swim across the English Channel). Instead, not knowing when I would adventure, I implemented a long, sport (swimming) specific *Base Mesocycle*. By doing this it would ensure I built:

- A large work capacity.
- Bulletproof resilience through strength training.
- A sizeable aerobic base ('gas tank').
- Specific Physical Preparedness for swimming.
- Strength and speed qualities for the sea through the Force-Velocity Curve.

Represented in a graph, my 2020 would look like this:

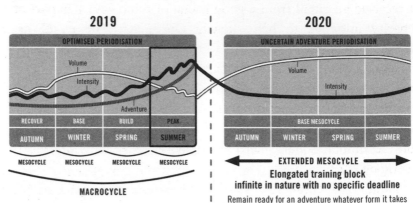

Living like a monk in isolation as England went in and out of various degrees of lockdown during the pandemic, I would follow the same daily routine as shown here.

MORNING	AFTERNOON	EVENING	NIGHT
10 km swim to improve aerobic fitness ('gas tank') and develop Specific Physical Preparedness.	Supplementary strength training to improve strength and speed qualities for swimming.	(Optional) Interval training to improve anaerobic fitness ('jet engine afterburners').	Research rivers, seas and swims.

The research bit would often go late into the night. Surrounded by tidal charts, maps and sailing routes, I would often start my evening by searching for a 'swim of significance' but, in the process, would be led down a 'rabbit hole' of marine conservation research. Hours would pass and many cups of cocoa would be drunk, until eventually I'd fall asleep on the sofa surrounded by pages of (often incoherent) notes.

But on 5 December 2020, it was different . . .

Somewhere between midnight and my sixth cup of hot chocolate, I received an email from a good friend of mine who was part of a charity initiative to help 'Rewild Our Seas'. The email itself contained a document that was 100 pages long and comprehensively detailed a three-year joint campaign between Parley (the collaborative that raises awareness for our oceans) and Talisker (the whisky distillery and manufacturer) that aimed to return the seas to the way they should be by supporting the preservation and protection of 100 million square metres of marine ecosystems around the world by 2023.

Now, I must confess I am a swimmer of oceans and not a scientist of seas, therefore (at the time) I didn't fully understand just how ambitious and important this project was. But as I continued to read (and brew more cocoa) I stumbled across the first ever systematic analysis of Earth's marine wilderness areas.[1] Within it, researchers aimed to identify places that are free from intense human impact, such as various types of fishing activity, commercial shipping, chemical run-off and climate change to name but a few. Shockingly, the study revealed was only 13.2 per cent of our oceans are now unspoiled and untouched as human activity threatens biodiversity and the functioning of marine ecosystems. The study concluded with clear instructions (and calls to action) addressed to political leaders, stating, 'Proactive retention of marine wilderness should now be incorporated into global strategies aimed at conserving biodiversity and ensuring that large-scale ecological and evolutionary processes continue.'

Similarly, around the same time world-renowned environmentalist Sir David Attenborough took to social media to single-handedly broadcast to his millions of followers that, 'Continents are on fire, glaciers are melting, coral reefs are dying and fish are disappearing from our oceans' and demanded world leaders act now, before it's too late. He added that the issues facing our planet are a 'communication issue as much as it is a scientific one' and demanded the public are made aware of the devastation and destruction.

Now at the risk of stating the obvious, I'm not a political leader.

No, I'm a swimmer who was reading this report while sitting in his pyjamas and slippers by his newly decorated Christmas tree. Therefore, logic would dictate that this 'call to arms' from Sir David Attenborough and marine biologists was not really addressed to me. But sleep-deprived, wired on cocoa beans and clearly not thinking straight, I had an idea and my thought process went a little something like this:

- In 2018, the Great British Swim was seen by 4 million viewers. It encouraged lots of people to get into open-water swimming.
- In 2019, the (attempted) swim across the English Channel was seen by 2 million people. It raised thousands of pounds for cancer research.

Therefore, I reasoned, what if in 2020 I made a 'swimming spectacle' of myself and attempted to swim really fast or really far across kelp forests, coral reefs and areas of marine wilderness to raise awareness for ocean conservation?

It was brilliant. The perfect formula for any adventure – askēsis in the pursuit of eudaimonia – and after exchanging several (late night) emails with my friends at Talisker and Parley, it was clear they thought so too and told me they had a support boat (and willing team) on the south coast of England who could help. Our only issue was that we needed to decide on the exact parameters of the swim. Would I be swimming to a headland? Around an island? Or between beaches?

The honest answer was, I didn't know. Which is why I fell asleep on the sofa that night content that I had a basic idea for an adventure, but concerned I had no specific details.

But I didn't need to worry.

In all my years of researching the science and psychology of adventure, I've found that sometimes you don't find the adventure. No, sometimes the adventure finds you. Whether it comes in the form of a particular mountain peak you feel innately drawn to climb, or an ocean crossing that's calling your name, there are some expeditions that just occur purely organically. And that's what happened the next morning when an idea for an aquatic adventure was delivered to me in the most unexpected way, from the most unlikely messenger.

SWIM TO FIND A SOLUTION

It was 7.30 a.m. on 6 December 2020 at Manley Mere, the morning after my night of marine research. Walking to the water's edge I was tightening my trunks and adjusting my goggles as I prepared for my daily 10 km swim. But I won't lie, starting today's session was harder than usual and I struggled to take off my warm hoodie and woollen trousers, since I knew the water waiting for me that day wasn't much warmer than 3°C (37.4°F). We were approaching the winter solstice (the shortest day of the year) when there's only eight hours of daylight. This meant my body's biological clock (circadian rhythm) was still having trouble grappling with the idea of starting to swim before the sun had fully risen in the sky. My clothes that day were slowly and reluctantly taken off and placed into my backpack and I stood there (in my trunks) stalling before my swim.

Looking around the lake at the local wildlife, I could see I wasn't the only one finding it hard to adapt to the longer nights and shorter days either. Owls overhead returned to their trees after a busy night's work and foxes rushed to find refuge among the dense trees and bushes. But as I sat there watching night turn to day, I accidentally bore witness to one of the most heroic races I've ever seen. An epic battle for the ages. It was Nature *v* Beast in its most powerful

279

and primitive form, as a tiny hedgehog went toe-to-toe with the rising sun and sprinted for cover, hoping to make it to the bushes and shrubbery before his cover was blown by the incoming sunrise that threatened to illuminate the entire lake.

Now, when I say 'sprinted' I mean it was quick for a hedgehog. I'm not a wildlife expert, but I imagine they're not renowned for their speed. But what this one lacked in raw pace, it made up for in grit and determination. With every minute that passed the shadows (and places to hide) disappeared, but refusing to accept defeat he swerved in and out of the long grass.

Why was he in such a hurry? Well, because the sunrise wasn't his only enemy. No, here on the battlefield that was Manley Mere he must also watch out for badgers on the ground and owls in the air. Two larger, angrier predators that the hedgehog knew he wouldn't stand a chance against in an old-fashioned fist fight should their paths cross, but concealed by the cover of darkness he could use his stealthy, night-time ninja skills to avoid such confrontations.

A few minutes passed and I was now so invested in the hedgehog's safety that I'd decided to temporarily postpone my swim. Still standing there in my trunks, I watched on with bated breath since I could see it had run out of grass and darkness to hide in. No longer able to sneak back home to the bushes, he had reached a kind of 'sunrise stalemate'. Out of time and out of options, he now had no choice but to boldly and bravely sprint across the open field where he'd be completely vulnerable to an attack from the owls above or the badgers below.

Peeking from behind his now poorly concealing patch of grass, I could see he was plucking up the courage to begin his run. That's because the field he had to cross to find safety was perhaps 800 metres long and although this might not sound like a lot, to a hedgehog it's practically an ultra-marathon. With a final check of the sky, sun and his surroundings, he looked left . . . he looked right . . . and then he was off.

As he did, the owls overhead among the trees began to stir and to sense breakfast could be served. But by this point, I was too involved in the success and survival of the hedgehog. I could no longer just spectate. With no time to get dressed again, I began sprinting across the field in my trunks trying to offer some form of defensive 'cover' for my spiky friend.

Watching on, I could see the owls were now questioning their airstrike too. Although the hedgehog looked appetising, they didn't know what to make of his larger, semi-naked friend running along-side him. Also, if there was a badger lurking in the grass, they'd likely be confused by the goggles still on my head and wonder why this strange, naked, beast had four eyes.

With 50 metres left I continued to operate as an offensive guard but now sensed the finish line was in sight and my tiny friend's battle with the sunrise, badgers and owls would be over. Celebrating, I cheered and gestured to him to stage a sprint finish as he ran into the dense woodland and disappeared down a burrow to his little hedgehog home.

Now I know what you're thinking, this is an odd way to spend a Sunday. Also, yes, I'm aware this wasn't normal behaviour for a 35-year-old man. But as I began my walk back across the field to the lake to resume my morning swim, I started to process what I'd just seen. In many ways, it was the purest form of race in the entire animal kingdom. It was sport against the sun. A duel that takes place between night and day. In that moment, I had an epiphany only explorers would understand and had an idea for my 'swim of significance' . . .

I would swim against the sun.

It would be the ultimate swimming spectacle. Approaching the winter solstice, I would jump into the sea when the sun rises, in water colder than 10°C (50°F) and would have around seven hours to swim as far as possible and as fast as possible. If the speed, distance or any metric of this swim was even remotely impressive, it could serve to raise awareness for ocean conservation and help the 'communication issue' facing our planet.

Messaging my friends at Talisker and Parley, I told them about the hedgehog, the idea and the swim against the sun. Needless to say, they loved it as much as I did. So, on 11 December 2020 boats were booked, captains were recruited and I headed to the south coast of England in search of askēsis at sea and my 'swim of significance'.

PART 4 | WHERE TO ADVENTURE

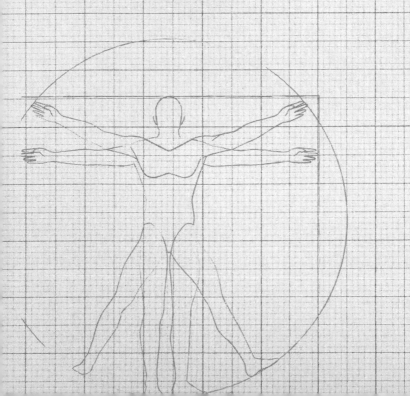

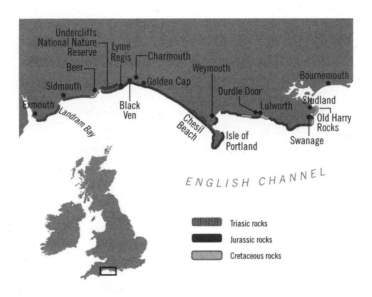

Triasic rocks
Jurassic rocks
Cretaceous rocks

LOCATION: *Dorset, England*
PROJECT: *Swim Against the Sun*
WATER TEMPERATURE: *9°C*

It was approaching midnight on 11 December 2020 as we arrived on the south coast of England in the county of Dorset after a 250-mile road trip. Known as the Jurassic Coast, because it's geological history can be traced back 185 million years, this area is a World Heritage Site renowned for its unique rock formations and stretches for 96 miles (154 km) down the coastline. In many ways, this would serve as the perfect 'race track' for our Swim Against the Sun.

But this particular December, during a COVID-19 pandemic, it was a very different story and nowhere was this more apparent than in the coastal town of Weymouth. Our temporary HQ for the swim, it's traditionally very popular with tourists as people travel from all over the country to visit its famous seafood festival, nearby castles and award-winning beaches. But tonight, this historic harbour was a cold, bleak, barren shadow of its former self as shops and restaurants were forced to shut. Even the marina itself was unrecognisable as the Weymouth and Portland National Sailing Academy, which previously hosted the sailing events of the 2012 Olympic Games, was void of its usual fleet of boats, ferries and private yachts.

But I didn't mind. I'm not a tourist or a sailor. No, I'm a swimmer who arrived at the quaint and semi-derelict seaside hotel we'd booked to meet the small, specialist team of individuals that Talisker and Parley had assembled for my Swim Against the Sun. Arriving from all over England, this crew uniquely comprised fearless filmmakers, skilled sailors and a very supportive girlfriend who each believed in the campaign as much as I did.

The latter was of course very important. That's because Hester had been my girlfriend for over eight years and supported me through so many sea swims around the world. Enduring sharks, storms and seasickness from Scotland to St Lucia, she's probably treated more jellyfish stings than any other girlfriend in history. Upon arrival, she immediately huddled around the table with the rest of the team to cross-reference maps and tidal charts with the waves and weather reports to decide the best day to embark on our aquatic adventure.

Looking around the room there were 10 of us in total, but the two most valued members of the team were Nick and Steve. Two captains who'd volunteered their services (and boats) to our cause and two sailing/diving hybrids who'd spent decades exploring the Dorset coastline (both above and below the water). Basically, they knew every shipwreck and coral reef in a 100 mile radius, so when they began to worry when looking at the reports . . . we *all* began to worry.

'What's wrong?' I asked concerned.

'There's a storm brewing,' Nick said. 'When it arrives, swimming and sailing will change from being difficult to semi-suicidal and it would be irresponsible of me as a captain to even leave the harbour.'

A sense of disappointment now filled the room as Steve explained how the south Dorset coast was famous for its shipwrecks as many captains throughout the centuries had fatally failed to respect the sea around these parts. Like a graveyard for boats, he told us over 1,000 sunken vessels now lay at the bottom of the seabed. Perhaps the most famous is the *Earl of Abergavenny*, one of the largest and most prestigious ships in the East India Company which had sailed across the globe to India (1797) and China (1798) and was even involved in the Napoleonic War (1804). But despite the impressive resume and miles of seafaring experience, the 177 ft ship sunk off the coast of Weymouth during a storm in February 1805, her 261 crew members perishing in the freezing water.

We all sat there in silence thinking over our options. Nick and Steve looked pensive as their eyes scanned every cliff, headland and bay on the Jurassic Coast.

'Can I make a suggestion?' Nick said.

'Yes,' I replied, trying to remain optimistic.

'What if we play "hide and seek" with the storm?'

Our joint disappointment now turned to collective confusion, but drawing on the map Nick was able to explain how we could use the shape of the shore and topography of the coastline to start the swim in 'stealth mode' and avoid the wrath of the weather.

'At 8.10 a.m. the sun begins to rise and the tides begin to change. Once this happens the water will begin to powerfully flow from east to west which means you will be shot out of Old Harry Rocks like a cannon with 1.2 knots assisting you, all while the coastline offers protection from the storm, wind and waves coming in the opposite direction,' he said pointing to the very eastern edge of the Jurassic Coast where he proposed we start the swim.

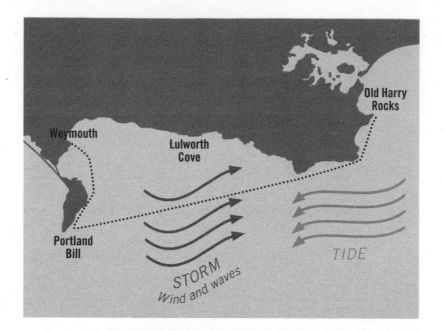

'But what happens when we swim around that headland, are no longer protected by the waves and the storm "finds us"?' Hester asked.

'I won't lie, it won't be pleasant,' Nick confessed.

He then explained how we'd have strong (spring) tides travelling in one direction and powerful winds pushing in the other. Known as 'wind over tide', it's where waves 'pile up' on top of each other, which means it would be like sailing (and swimming) in white water rapids as you get battered by the sea from sunrise to sunset.

'Basically, it will be less about swimming and more about surviving. But if you're strong enough to remain above the water, and not below it, you'll be pushed over 40 to 50 km towards Portland Bill and Weymouth where you can hide from the storm again and be protected by the coastline during sunset.'

Looking at the map, I took a moment to process the plan, since I knew this wouldn't be a swim in the traditional sense. Instead, I'd be trying to 'ride the tide' as I got beaten, battered and bruised by the wind, waves and weather. But we had an ocean conservation campaign to launch and 100 million square metres of vital marine ecosystems to protect. Plus, to quote Franklin D Roosevelt, 'A smooth sea never made a skilled sailor [or swimmer]' and in many ways, this would be the perfect proving ground for every theory written in this book. Attempting to swim as far as possible, as fast as possible, the following questions would be answered:

- Had I drilled Specific Physical Preparedness for the ocean?
- Did I have a big enough aerobic base ('gas tank')?
- Was I anaerobically capable of swimming at higher intensities ('jet engine afterburners')?
- Had I developed strength and speed qualities for the sea through the Force-Velocity Curve?

Essentially, if I failed the theories contained within these chapters were wrong. But if I succeeded, this book would become a proven blueprint for anyone wanting to know *How to Adventure*. Hoping it would be the latter, I turned to the team.

'I want to swim, but understand if you don't,' I said.

I knew sea swimming was not an individual sport and this particular swim would require the unwavering support of a crew who'd have to sail under constant threat of a storm. But what happened next, I will never forget. Barely a word was spoken. Instead, maps were folded away, laptops were closed and alarms were set as a group of complete strangers agreed to meet at the harbour at 6 a.m., in complete darkness, to start a swim against the sun . . . and a game of 'hide and seek' against a storm.

SWIM FROM THE SUN, HIDE FROM THE STORM

The time was 7.52 a.m. and we had arrived at the start line for our race against the sun. With 'battle plans' finalised with the safety crew, I decided to perch myself on the side of the boat to make adjustments to my wetsuit. It was a new prototype I was testing that came with extra zips, buttons and flaps that made it easier to get on, adjust and visit the toilet when nature called. It also had an inbuilt thermometer in the sleeve which I was currently using to take a temperature reading. Submerging it in the water, I already knew my swim would be far from tropical, but a reading of 8.1°C (46.6°F) confirmed that the day would be particularly uncomfortable.

But this was typical of the British sea in winter. It almost had a menacing and mischievous quality to it that made even the most hardened sailors long for the safety and sanctuary of the marina. However, any thoughts of warmth and wellbeing would have to wait since our highly anticipated sunrise was now almost upon us and our team of filmmakers and photographers was determined to capture it in all its glory. With their lifejackets tightly fastened and cameras perfectly poised, they'd been told the sunrises over this part of the coast were legendary and so were committed to capturing the very moment the sun rose out of the sea and signalled the start of our swim.

No-one, however, was more committed than our team's director. Poised at the helm of the boat, he'd produced environmental media projects around the world, from rhino protection in South Africa to combating deforestation in Borneo. Basically, he was as professional as he was passionate, and like a Spielberg of the sea he had a romantic vision of how he wanted our swim against the sun to unfold.

'Everyone ready?' his voice reverberated around the boat.

The team nodded in unison and I put my goggles on.

'Three, two, one . . . GO!' he shouted, as the first beam of light illuminated the cliffs.

Leaping from the boat and diving headfirst into the water, I was so keen to stage the epic start to the swim that everyone wanted. Unfortunately, I was completely unaware a zip had broken on my wetsuit at the most unfortunate time, in the most unfortunate position. As a result, the media team started their day with a shot of me jumping into the water as my 'poo flap' whistled in the wind. Shouting from the boat, our director was far from happy.

'Ross! What was that?' he screamed.

'It's my prototype poo flap,' I replied. 'I think it's broken.'

With his head in his hands, it's clear he didn't have the time (or patience) for any wardrobe malfunctions in the script.

'Ross, let's try to remember, we're trying to inspire people to protect and preserve our oceans. I'm not sure footage of your poo flap helps to convey this message.'

He sounded genuinely angry, so I didn't want to tell him my flap needed fixing and that my left buttock was suffering from a strange form of 'cold shock'. Instead, I decided to keep quiet, swim and hope it warmed up in the rising sun.

This worked for a while and two hours into our seven-hour swim against the sun, I had temporarily forgotten about the faulty flap on

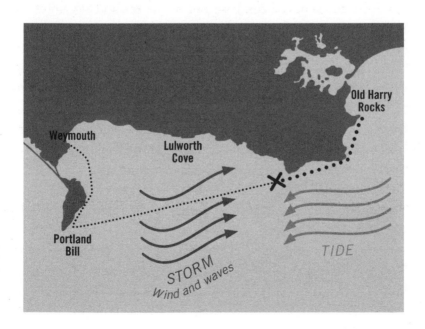

my wetsuit since progress was good and we'd covered over 15 km (9.3 miles). This was mainly thanks to the joint genius of Nick and Steve who'd predicted the tides perfectly, but was also because (as planned) the cliffs of the Jurassic Coast were offering some welcome protection from the wind and waves that continued to build up.

Of course, we knew it wouldn't all be smooth sailing. That's because as the storm we all feared continued to brew, we were about to swim around the most southerly part of the Purbeck peninsula (known as St Alban's Head). Once we did, we'd be entering 'no man's land' and would have to swim sprint 30 km to the Isle of Portland before we were offered any form of shelter and safety from the shape of the coastline.

Basically, frostbitten buttocks would be the least of my worries.

Turning the corner and as expected myself and the boat were immediately assaulted by waves. Travelling with such force and ferocity, they relentlessly tested the durability of our boat, the resilience of our stomachs and the strength of my rotator cuffs. Thankfully, after a year-long *Base Mesocycle* I had faith in my shoulders, but knew little could be done for the team who were being plagued by seasickness.

Within minutes the sea claimed its first victim. One of our assistant producers was being so violently sick that they'd gone from throwing up their breakfast to vomiting stomach bile. This is the greenish-yellow material made in your liver and stored in your gallbladder which you can throw up when you're so seasick that this is the only thing left in your stomach.

Looking up at the boat, it was hard to describe what I witnessed. But if you imagine a horror movie combined with a pirate film, you begin to get a rough idea. In fact, the only other time I'd seen seasickness like this was in the Caribbean during the 100 km swim from Martinique to St Lucia. The entire crew was so ill they couldn't swallow any seasick tablets without bringing them back up, so had to 'plug' them up their bums as a makeshift rectal suppository.

Does it work? Surprisingly, yes.

Was our seasick assistant producer going to try it? Not surprisingly, no.

It turns out this wasn't a seasick solution any of the team were willing to entertain. So Nick was forced to take the worst affected members of our crew back to shore, leaving Steve behind in a smaller support boat with our head of health and safety. But I didn't mind, since our head of safety was a modern-day seafaring Spartan. A former Royal Marine turned paramedic, Trevor (Smith) was a good friend of mine who I had previously worked with on a series of ice swimming adventures. Which explains why he was perfectly at home among storms at sea.

Trevor casually leant over the side of the boat (among crashing waves) to offer me a banana, electrolyte drink and malt loaf.

'How's everything going down there?' he enquired.

'Yes, fine. Why do you ask?'

'Well, you've been in the water a few hours now and your lips are looking a little blue,' he said.

I then told him about the faulty flap on my wetsuit and how I was losing heat through my left buttock. Trevor understandably looked confused. As a paramedic with years of experience managing expeditions all over the world, he thought he'd heard it all. But he confessed this was a unique problem that he'd never come across before.

'Hmm . . . we've another 5 hours and 35 km (21.7 miles) to swim. That's a long time to be in water of 8.1°C (46.6°F), so I'm going to need you to talk to me as clearly and as frequently as possible,' he said, knowing that any signs of slurred speech, confusion and an inability to communicate would be an early indication of hypothermia.

I nodded and understood, but this was easier said than done.

Over the next few hours the waves became angrier, my body felt colder and my lips turned another shade of blue. As a result, convincing Trevor that I was okay was proving tricky as I battled two new enemies in the form of cold diuresis and low muscle glycogen.

Firstly, cold diuresis[1] is the strong (sometimes uncontrollable) desire to urinate that can happen as your body reacts to cold temperatures. It does this since the body starts to constrict your blood vessels (known as vasoconstriction) to reduce blood flow to the skin and keep the warmth around your internal organs. This in turn causes an increase in blood pressure because there is now the same amount of blood in your body being pumped through a smaller amount of space. In response to this increase in pressure, the kidneys begin to filter out excess fluid in the blood to reduce the blood's volume, and therefore the pressure. Of course, all this fluid has to go somewhere, which explains why I'd been urinating non-stop since Old Harry Rocks and stopping every 30 minutes to combat this perpetual mechanism of dehydration that plagues marathon swimmers.

But dehydration wasn't my only concern.

Ever since I had swum beyond the protective headland, I had been forced to battle huge waves and operate at a higher intensity. This meant I had switched from relying on my aerobic energy system ('gas tank') to my anaerobic energy system ('jet engine afterburners') and was now burning through muscle glycogen (the body's stored form of carbohydrates) at a rate of knots in order to produce energy and 'power' the body (adenosine triphosphate). This was no longer just a swim against the sun or a game of 'hide and seek' against a storm. No, it was an eating competition as I tried to consume carbohydrates as fast as I was burning through them.

Of course, for years we've known that, 'Dietary carbohydrate loading[2] improves endurance,'[3] and that, 'Muscle glycogen[4] [carbohydrate] availability can affect performance,'[5] but very few studies have been done on salty bananas, flapjacks and sweets at sea while battling the cold. Which explains why, with 35 km (21.7 miles)

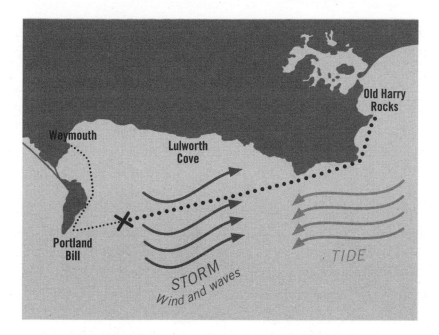

covered and Portland Bill lighthouse now firmly in our sights, the following conversation with Trevor and Steve was a strange one that only adventurers would understand.

'You look like you're getting worse,' Trevor said as he passed me a banana.

'No, no . . . I'm fine,' I said, struggling to talk as my lips were now frozen shut from the cold.

Trevor looked down on me from the boat with concern. Frowning, he watched on as I ate and shook his head since I couldn't actually chew the food he was giving me and instead was just trying to place it in and around my mouth in the hope some of it would be swallowed and ingested.

'Hmm . . . you're urinating and dribbling a lot for someone who claims they're fine,' he said.

He then explained how finishing this swim (and making it back to Weymouth) could go from being difficult to outright dangerous for two reasons:

- BREATHING BECOMES HARDER. Studies show an adventurer's aerobic capacity (the ability of the heart and lungs to get oxygen to the muscles) falls in relation to my body temperature.[6] According to research from the *Journal of Applied Physiology*, a 0.5°C fall in core temperature can result in a 10–30 per cent fall in VO2 max (lung capacity) and maximum cardiac output (the volume of blood being pumped by the heart).[7]

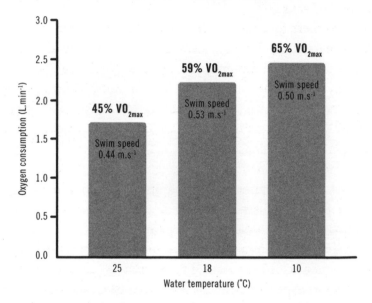

Mean oxygen consumption during 90-minute swims in different water temperatures. The increase in oxygen consumption when swimming in colder water is due to the super-imposition of shivering on swimming metabolism.[8]

- LIMBS FEEL HEAVIER. The limbs have a high surface-area-to-mass ratio so are greatly impacted by the cold[9] as the muscles' ability to move and contract (contractile force) is significantly impaired when its temperature falls below 27°C. According to an article published in *Aviation Space and Environmental Medicine* this is, 'Due to factors such as reduced enzyme activity, decreased acetylcholine and calcium release, slower rates of diffusion and decreased muscle perfusion.'[10]

Back on the boat, Steve was equally worried. He was looking at the sun in the sky and the watch on his arm.

'It's been a great swim, Ross. There would be no shame in stopping now,' he said.

I floated there for a moment knowing they were both right.

From years of coaching sea swimming, I knew my body was shutting down from cold diuresis, low muscle glycogen and now early signs of hypothermia. I also knew that swimming 35 km against the sun in water temperatures as low as 8.1°C (46.6°F) with a broken 'poo flap' is a noble swim and valiant effort that would help raise awareness for ocean conservation.

But that is not *How to Adventure*. No, from years of studying I knew that great happiness can be found in extreme hardship and that a deep, personal sense of eudaimonia would only be found if I was to swim back into Weymouth Harbour.

As my body's core temperature dropped below 35°C and I battled the subsequent confusion and disorientation, I thought about the years of sports-specific, Spartan-inspired askēsis and instead chose to ignore my bladder, broken 'poo flap', dwindling energy reserves and impaired lung capacity. Then, one stroke at a time, I headed towards Weymouth with a dogged but determined technique under the watchful eye of Trevor and Steve as the sun began to set in the sky.

Did it work? Well, to this day I'm not sure I believe in symbolism or not, but the final hour of our swim was performed under the most incredible sunset as two dolphins joined me for the last 10 km of the swim back into Weymouth Harbour. Circling our support boat and swimming under me, (I was later told) dolphins in Celtic culture are seen as protectors which is why I like to think maybe (just maybe) they knew what we were doing there that day and wanted to help. Either that or they were wondering why this odd human had a broken 'poo flap', had a banana in his beard and strongly smelt of urine.

Moments later, I emerged from the water in the marina. The final distance I had swum was 53 km (32.9 miles), in 7 hours and 11 minutes. Reuniting with the rest of the team, celebratory drinks

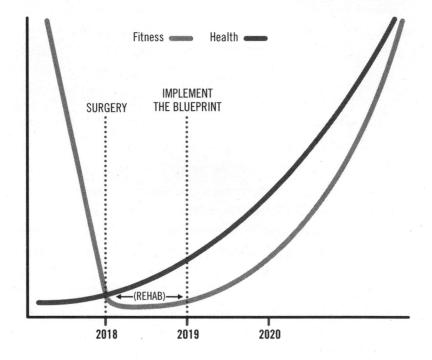

were then poured and a hot bath was run to help me recover before speaking to local journalists.

But as I sat there in the bath trying my best to defrost my left bum cheek and thaw out my face, I couldn't help but smile. Not because I was happy, but because I had achieved a profound sense of eudaimonia by following a *Blueprint* I created, inspired by Bruce Lee and LeBron

James and founded upon years of tried and tested sports science and ancient warrior philosophy. Going from surgery to sea, (as represented in the diagram below) I was no longer fatigued and sick, but fit and strong. My health and fitness now worked in perfect harmony as I built my body from the ground up and from the inside out.

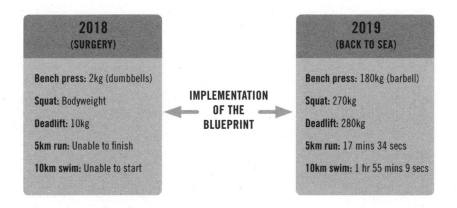

2018 (SURGERY)	IMPLEMENTATION OF THE BLUEPRINT	2019 (BACK TO SEA)
Bench press: 2kg (dumbbells)		**Bench press:** 180kg (barbell)
Squat: Bodyweight		**Squat:** 270kg
Deadlift: 10kg		**Deadlift:** 280kg
5km run: Unable to finish		**5km run:** 17 mins 34 secs
10km swim: Unable to start		**10km swim:** 1 hr 55 mins 9 secs

This is why as the year 2020 came to an end, I wouldn't necessarily say I had matured. Since I'm still the same guy with a broken 'poo flap' on his urine-soaked wetsuit who ran across a field semi-naked to protect a hedgehog. But from 2018 to 2020, I would claim I had aged and evolved and learnt to:

Turn wounds into wisdom,
Scars into strength,
And injuries into intelligence.

Now, looking ahead to 2021, I had no idea what adventures awaited me since travel was still uncertain in the midst of a global pandemic, but that's okay. That's also the very nature of being an explorer as the mountains, oceans and jungles are entirely unpredictable and the weather, waves and seasons completely untameable. But the beauty of this book is that for me (and anyone reading it) it provides proven sports science principles (arranged in a systematic way) to prepare for you for any expedition. Written to become a blueprint for anyone wanting to know *How to Adventure*, it's my hope this book:

- Becomes an essential item for any explorer's backpack or bookcase.
- Ushers in a new era of athletic adventures.
- Brings the science and psychology of adventure into the twenty-first century.

But most importantly, I hope the stories found throughout these pages have made you smile, the workouts have enriched your training and the teachings have inspired you to find a map, form a plan and embark on some incredible (truly eudaimonic) adventures of your own.

EXERCISES | COACHING CUES

'PULL' TRAINING EXERCISES

Passive Hang (Brachiating)

Grab onto a bar or support system with a slightly wider-than-shoulder width grip, palms facing away. Be sure to wrap your all fingers around the bar, with your thumb also wrapped (called the full grip). Once you have secured yourself to the bar, allow yourself to hang without your feet touching the ground. Be sure to keep your spine in alignment, limiting any upper back rounding and lower back extension. You should start to feel a stretch across the upper back, armpits and maybe even biceps/triceps. Try to keep the head and neck relaxed so that the ears sit slightly in front of the biceps. Allow the weight of the body to stretch the muscles deeper, being sure to always make mental checks to stay aware of spinal positioning and body tension (so, try to relax instead of tensing up).

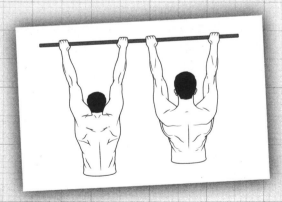

Dynamic Hanging

There are multiple dynamic hang variations. For the side-to-side one, start swinging by lifting one leg and hip up towards the ribs on the same side, dropping back toward the centre and repeating fluidly from left to right. Once you're swinging to the side, release the weightless hand at the top of your swing and then re-catch it. Repeat on the other side, trying to keep your shoulders active but not tense. Keep the shoulders blades back and down and ribcage down.

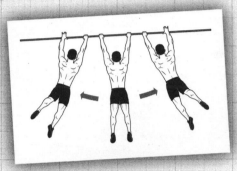

Scapula Pull-Ups

Grip the pull-up bar with both hands. Your hands should be slightly wider than shoulder-width distance apart and your palms should be facing away from you. Hang from the bar and enter a passive hang with the shoulders relaxed. Without bending your arms or swinging, perform a reverse shrug to depress your shoulder blades. Pause for a second at the bottom, then return your shoulders to the starting position.

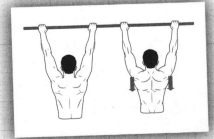

Overhead Medicine Ball Slams

Stand with feet hip width apart, knees slightly bent and hold the medicine ball with two hands directly overhead. Slam the ball to the ground in front of you as hard as you can, engaging your abs and glutes while paying particular attention to engage the large muscles of the back (latissimus dorsi) which are used when swimming. Then pick the ball up, raise overhead and repeat for desired number of repetitions ensuring you train within the Peak Power and Speed-Strength Training Zone of the Force-Velocity Curve.

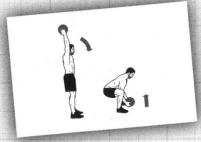

Pull-Ups (pronated) (Optional: Weighted)

Grip the bar with your hands shoulder width apart and your palms facing away from you. Hang with your arms fully extended and keep your shoulders back and your core engaged. Then pull yourself up until your chin passes the bar until slowly lowering yourself down until your arms are extended again.

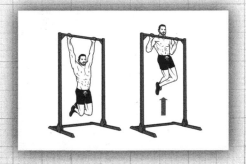

303

Underhand (supinated) Close-Grip Pull-Ups (Optional: Weighted)

Grasp a pull-up bar with an underhand grip, hands shoulder-width apart or slightly narrower. Straighten your arms, keep your knees bent and cross your lower legs. Retract your shoulder blades to reduce the stress on the shoulder joints. Keeping your body stable and core engaged, pull your body up until your chin becomes aligned with the bar. Pause for one to two seconds at the top, with the biceps under maximum tension. Slowly lower to the start position.

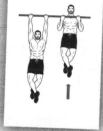

Single-Arm Dumbbell Row

You need a bench or a sturdy thigh-high platform to lean on when doing the exercise, so secure that first and place a dumbbell on the floor to one side of it. Put your left leg on the bench and grab the far side with your left hand, then bend over so your upper body is parallel with the ground. Reach down and pick up the dumbbell in your right hand with a neutral grip (palm facing you), then hold it with your arm extended, keeping your back straight. Bring the dumbbell up to your chest, concentrating on lifting it with your back and shoulder muscles rather than your arms. Keep your chest still as you lift. At the top of the movement, squeeze your shoulder and back muscles. Lower the dumbbell slowly until your arm is fully extended again. Do all your reps on one arm before switching to the other side.

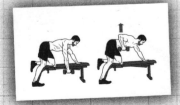

Spider Bicep Curls

Grab a dumbbell in each hand and position yourself lying face first on an inclined bench. Then extend your biceps down and out in front of you. Then contract your biceps and curl the weights up towards your shoulders, squeezing your muscles in the process and isolating the biceps. Hold for a count when you reach the top position then return back to the starting position.

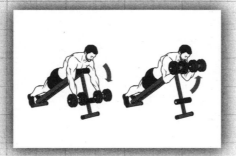

Rope Pulls

Attach the rope to a sled, kettlebell or anything that can be dragged. Grasp the rope at the opposite end in preparation for the drag. Straddle the rope with both legs. Your feet should be wider than shoulder width apart. Begin pulling the rope. Your waist should be bent and the pulling should take place at the hip level or below. Knees should be bent approximately 90 degrees. Continue the drag until you run out of rope.

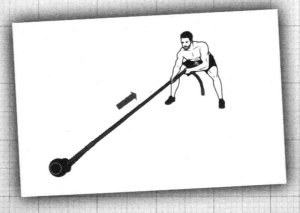

305

Farmer's Walk

Stand between two sets of weights—dumbbells, kettlebells or custom barbells. Place your hands in the middle of the weights to avoid tipping them. Brace your core and glutes and drive through the floor to lift the weights. Straighten your posture, get tall, look straight ahead. Take small, quick steps for the allotted distance or time. Put the weights down in a controlled manner.

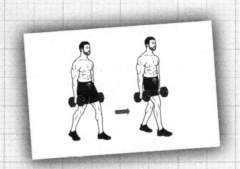

Hanging Barbell High Pull

The high pull hits your mid-back, rhomboids and rear delts (as well as the whole posterior chain: hamstrings, glutes and lower back). The lift starts with the barbell at mid-thigh (or from the blocks), with the shoulders slightly forward of the line of the bar and the neck in a neutral position. The shoulder blades are pulled together and the chest is as high as possible to allow for proper stability of the upper back, thus providing the optimal environment for the highest power output. At this point, start pulling as high as possible towards the neck using the posterior chain muscles and keeping the bar close to the body for all of the duration of the lift. Once the full extension of the legs and hips is reached, actively shrug and continue pulling the elbows high and to the sides to allow the upper arms to reach a horizontal position, parallel to the floor.

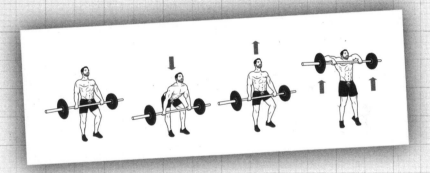

Cable Face Pulls

This exercise is performed to restore balance within the shoulder joint to prevent injuries. Using a cable machine, grab the ends of the rope and take a few steps back, so you are leaning backward slightly and looking up at the pulley. Keeping your elbows up, pull the rope back, towards the top of your head, pinching your shoulder blades together. Remaining in control, return the rope to starting position.

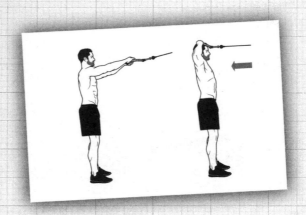

Band-Resisted Single-Arm Rows

Band-Resisted Single-Arm Rows are a great variation of the conventional single-arm dumbbell row because they create mechanical tension at the bottom of the dumbbell row where you'd normally allow your arms to just hang. The idea is to make you work through a greater range of motion to train both speed and strength. To do this variation I recommend performing banded dumbbell rows with 1) the band anchored directly above the shoulder of your rowing arm when you're in the bent-over position to begin the row, and 2) around the top of your forearm, just below your elbow.

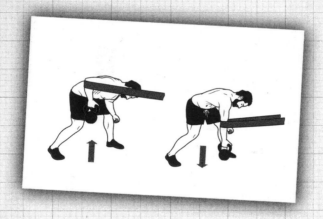

Single-Arm Plank Rope Pulls

Blending two motions (a plank and a single-arm pull-up) into one, this unilateral movement (single limb) engages the core and replicates the coordinated, unilateral (single arm), cross-body muscle connection needed in swimming. To perform this, get in a forearm plank position, with the rope between your arms. You should be as far from the sled as possible. Reach in front to pick up the rope with one hand, maintaining the plank position. Squeeze your glutes and keep your hips steady. Pull the sled in towards yourself, keeping your torso facing the ground. Make sure to keep the arm you're pulling with tight to your body and avoid flaring your elbow out; think of it as a fully vertical movement, like a pull-up. Continue pulling until you bring the sled all the way in. Reposition the rope and repeat with the other arm.

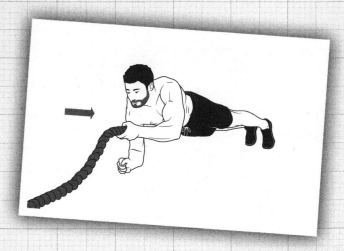

LOWER-BODY & LEG EXERCISES

Front Seated Squats

The front squat is a variation of the conventional squat that places a greater emphasis on the core. To perform this movement, step up to the rack and rest the bar on your upper chest (close to your neck, but not touching). Elbow placement and grip are key. Place your fingers under the bar, so the elbows lift forward, up and away from the body (hands placed shoulder-width apart). Try to get your elbows up to bar height throughout this move. With a good upright spinal position un-rack the bar and place feet a bit wider than hip-distance apart with toes pointed out slightly. Begin to lower the body into a squat. Keep the spine long and upright. Your hips stay under the bar (rather than floating behind the bar in a traditional squat). Try not to shift forward onto the balls of the feet or back into the heels. At the lowest position, your hamstrings will nearly touch the back of the calves (elbows still lifted at bar height and chest upright). Lift out of the squat in a slow, controlled manner with the hips and knees extending simultaneously. Continue lifting until the body is back at the starting position.

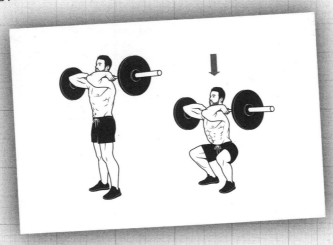

Seated (Box) Squats

Stand with your feet shoulder-width apart in front of a box with a loaded barbell resting on the back of your shoulders. Push your hips back, and bend at the knees to get into a half-squat position. Descend into a full squat position, but be sure not to sit on the box top. Pause when thighs are parallel and just a few inches from the box top. Brace core, pause, and then drive hips upward back into starting position.

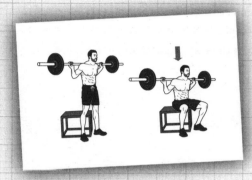

(Dumbbell) Weighted Lunges

Stand with your torso upright holding 2 dumbbells in your hands by your sides. Take a big step forward with right leg and start to shift weight forward so heel hits the floor first. Lower body until right thigh is parallel to floor and right shin is vertical (it's okay if knee shifts forward a little as long as it doesn't go past right toe). If mobility allows, lightly tap left knee to ground while keeping weight in right heel. Press into right heel to drive back up to starting position. Repeat on the other side.

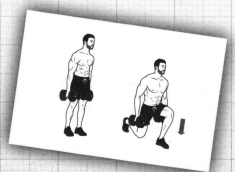

Barbell Standing Barefoot Calf (Toe) Raises

Calf raises are a great replication of the propulsive phase of running, but performing them barefoot is a good way of improving proprioception which teaches us to drive off the big toe with efficient running biomechanics/technique. Start by placing a block or two free weight plates on the floor, then placing a weighted barbell across your back and step up so that the balls of your feet are on the block. Driving specifically through the big toe, slowly lift your heels up off of the floor and then lower them back so that you feel as much of a stretch as possible in your calf muscles. Return to the starting position and repeat.

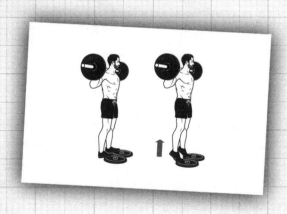

(Barbell) Reverse Lunges

Place the barbell on your back and take a large and controlled step backward with your left foot. Lower your hips so that your right thigh (front leg) becomes parallel to the floor with your right knee positioned directly over your ankle. Your left knee should be bent at a 90-degree angle and pointing toward the floor with your left heel lifted. Return to standing by pressing your right heel into the floor and bringing your left leg forward to complete one rep. Alternate legs, and step back with right leg.

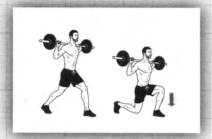

Single-Arm Overhead Kettlebell Lunge

A lunge progression that requires a greater degree of coordination and balance. Hold a single kettlebell overhead and keep the weight directly in line with the shoulder joint. Step out with the opposite leg. Once the foot touches the ground, drop the hips toward the deck keeping the knee behind the toe. Pushing through the heel power back up to the start position.

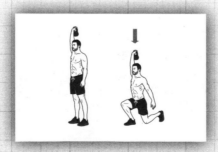

Prowler Push

The prowler push is very simple to perform and requires very little training since it's a natural movement. But ensure your arms extended (high-grip) and keep your body at around a 45-degree angle. Also ensure your face is pointing to the ground, your neck aligned with your back.

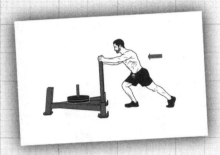

Box Jumps

Stand in front of the box with feet directly under the hips and hands by your side. Lower yourself into the jumping position by bending at the knees and hips. Keep your head up and back straight. Explosively jump from the crouched position while swinging the arms. Land softly on the centre of the platform absorbing the impact with your legs. Stand tall. Return to starting position by stepping down and repeat the movement.

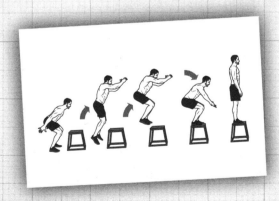

Single-Arm Dumbbell Side Lunge and Touch

A brilliant contralateral, unilateral, full-body exercise where one side of the body is kept long and stretched while the other side is short and contracted. The timing and counterbalance of the two can create significant power (like during a swim stroke). To perform this stand while holding a dumbbell in your right hand. Let it hang at arm's length by your side. Take a big step to your left and lower your body by pushing your hips backward and bending your left knee. As you lower your body, bend forward at your hips and touch the dumbbell to the floor on the inside of your left foot. You'll have to lean forward at your hips to do this, but focus on keeping your chest up, instead of allowing your torso to slump forward. If you can't touch the floor without rounding your lower back, only lower as far as you can while keeping your back naturally arched. Pause, and then push yourself back up to the starting position. That's 1 rep.

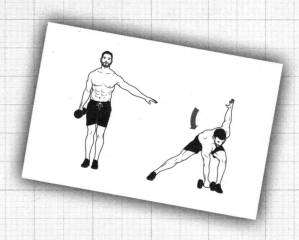

Battle Rope Wrestler Throws

Grab the ropes in a reverse grip so the ends are pointing towards the ceiling. Whip the ropes up and over, rotating your whole body to the left. Then whip up and over and rotate your whole body to the right. Do as many reps as you can, always imagining you're throwing the rope to the floor. The goal here is to improve hip rotation since many distance swimmers rely on their hip rotation to generate power and allow them to take longer and stronger strokes.

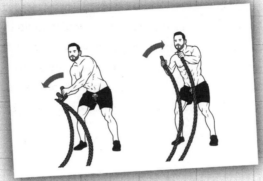

The Stability Ball Log roll

Get in a push-up position with the stability ball under your legs between your knees and feet position. Twist your body from the hip/torso area keeping your upper body from shifting too much. Twist as much as 90 degrees to the right and then to the left. Be sure to reposition the stability ball if it shifts out of place.

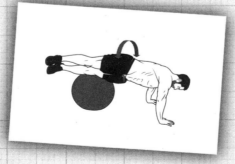

Pallof Hold and Press

The Pallof Hold and Press is a core stabilisation exercise. To do it, hold the band in both hands at mid-chest height, right around your solar plexus. Turn sideways, so the tension is coming across your body, and step laterally so you increase the tension on the cable/band. Inhale, then exhale as you fully straighten your arms in front of you. Hold there for at least two seconds – the longer you hold, the tougher it is – and inhale as you bend your elbow to bring your hands back in. Repeat.

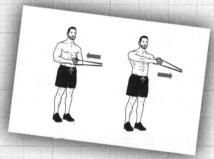

V-Sit Flutter Kick

This exercise is tough, as it will challenge your lower back, hip flexors as well as taxing your abs. To perform these sit on the ground and start 'fluttering your legs' up and down. Focus on making small kicks (mimicking your actual kicking action as closely as possible). Balance yourself with your hands if necessary by placing them on the floor, but if possible bring your arms above your head into a streamline position. Your body's natural inclination will be to roll backwards, but use your core to stabilise your body so that this doesn't occur.

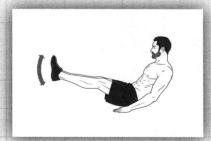

'PUSH' TRAINING EXERCISES

Scapula Push-Ups

Performed to strengthen the muscles around the scapula (specifically serratus anterior – when you strengthen it, you promote normal scapula motion and improve shoulder mobility). Start in a conventional push-up position (hands directly underneath your shoulders). Keep your body in a straight line and your head relaxed in a neutral position, aligned with the rest of your spine. Tighten your core and glute muscles so your hips don't sink. Keep your arms extended and pinch your shoulder blades together. Try to imagine pinching a pencil between your shoulder blades. Retract and protract your shoulder blades, lowering your body slightly. The range of motion is small. Do not lower your chest all the way to the floor. Hold each rep for 3–5 seconds. Release and return to a high plank position.

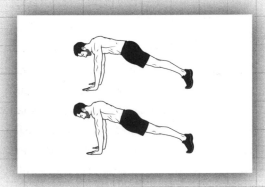

Internal Rotation with Band

This form of conditioning is similar to the external rotation exercise; however, this strengthens the subscapularis muscle. Stand with your side to the door, elbow at 90 degrees and the band tied to something stable. Now rotate your arm towards your body. Remember to keep those shoulder blades back and down throughout the entire movement.

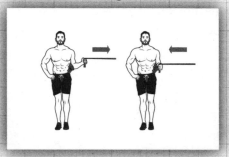

External Rotation with Band

This exercise is excellent for strengthening the external rotators and for general scapula stability. Use a relatively light resistant band and tie to something stable. Stand with your side to the door, place a towel underneath your arm and lock your elbow in by your side with it bent at 90 degrees. Now stand tall, while rotating your arm away from your body and then back to the starting position slowly. It is important that you maintain a good posture while doing this exercise, which means keeping your shoulder blades back and down throughout the entire movement.

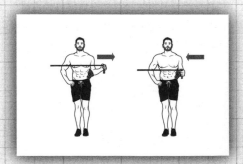

Plyometric Push-Ups

An advanced form of the conventional push-up. Assume a push-up position. Squeeze your glutes and brace your abs. Bend your elbows and lower your body until your chest nearly touches the floor. Then press yourself up so forcefully that your hands leave the floor. Clap your hands together before returning them to the floor. That's one rep. Another great alternative is a Single Arm Rotational Med Ball Throw which allows you train in the same Speed Strength Training Zone while also engaging the hips.

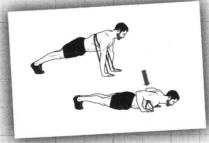

Band-Resisted Push-Ups

Hook your thumbs through a resistance band and loop the band behind your back. Assume a plank position with your hands on the floor so that they're slightly wider than your shoulders. Your body should form a straight line from your ankles to your head. Squeeze your glutes and brace your abdominals. Maintain this stability for the duration of the exercise. Lower your body until your chest nearly touches the floor. Pause at the bottom, and then push yourself back to the starting position.

Barbell Bench Press

Lie flat on your back on a bench. Grip the bar with hands just wider than shoulder-width apart, so when you're at the bottom of your move your hands are directly above your elbows. This allows for maximum force generation. Bring the bar slowly down to your chest as you breathe in. Push up as you breathe out, gripping the bar hard and watching a spot on the ceiling rather than the bar, so you can ensure it travels the same path every time.

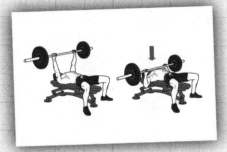

Dumbbell Shoulder Press

Sit on an upright bench holding a dumbbell in each hand at shoulder height with your palms facing away from you. Keep your chest up and your core braced, and look straight forward throughout the move. Press the weights directly upwards until your arms are straight and the weights touch above your head. Slowly lower the weights back to the start position under control, pause, then start the next rep.

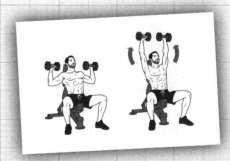

Single-Arm Kettlebell Shoulder Press

Very good for developing shoulder strength and stability within the joint it also works the entire body since the unilateral (one-sided) nature of the exercise forces you to engage the core like you would when swimming to remain in a streamlined position. To begin this exercise; start off by clean pressing a kettlebell to your shoulder with your palms facing inward towards your face. Then press the kettlebell up and out until it is overhead. Return the kettlebell back to the inward shoulder position and then repeat.

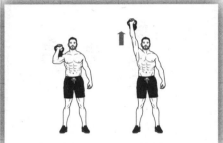

Tricep Pushdowns

Set the cable machine up with the bar at head height. Grab the bar, keep the back straight and your elbows tucked in. Stand with your feet hip-width apart. Pull the cable down until the bar touches your thighs and pause to squeeze your triceps at the bottom. Then slowly raise the bar back to the starting position. (This exercise can also be performed with a resistance band if you do not have access to a cable machine.)

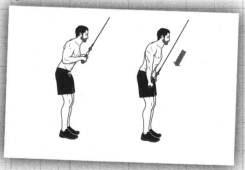

Standing Barbell Shoulder Press

The movement begins in the bottom (start) position. Stand with your entire body tight and rigid. Hold a barbell just above your upper chest, hands slightly wider that shoulder width. Now think of an imaginary straight line drawn from the elbows through the wrists and hands and into the ceiling. Press the bar up along this path as the elbows extend, taking the same path back down to the starting position.

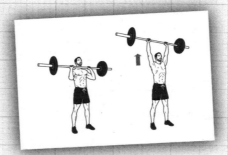

Ring Dips

Adjust the height of the rings so that your feet will not touch the ground between repetitions. Mount the rings and assume the support position. You should be above the rings, arms straight, supporting your body weight. Lower your body down by bending at the elbows and keeping shoulders close to your sides. Keep the movement steady and controlled. If possible, continue down until your shoulders almost touch your hands for a full range of motion. Press your body back to the original starting position.

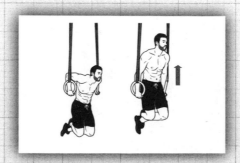

Bear Crawls

Get down on all fours, with your hands directly under your shoulders and your knees under your hips. Bring your knees off the ground and travel forward. Keep your back flat at all times. Travel 10 metres forward, then reverse.

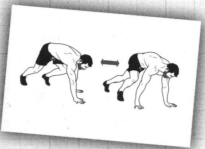

Band-Resisted Tricep Push-Downs

Band-Resisted Tricep Push-Downs are a variation of the standard tricep push-down that's performed on a cable machine. To start, attach (and 'anchor') your resistance band above your head and grab it with an overhand grip with your arms at the level of your sternum. Step back from the anchor point a couple of inches and bend at the waist so that your torso is at about a 45-degree angle to the floor. Now straighten your arm to perform a triceps push-down that more closely replicates the final part of a front crawl stroke (in the fully extended position, your hands should be slightly behind your body).

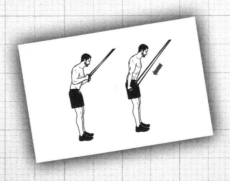

Battle Rope Plank Single-Arm Waves

Great for developing shoulder strength and stability within the joint and replicating the unilateral (one-sided) nature of swimming that forces you to engage the core like you would when swimming to remain in a streamlined position. Start in the plank position with your abs fully engaged and your body straight. Hold the rope in your right hand and raise your left leg. Wave your right hand up and down, keeping the rest of your body stable, for 15 seconds, then switch sides and repeat. Rest for 30 seconds and repeat five times.

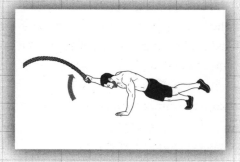

STRONGMAN SESSION EXERCISES

Sledgehammers

Stand in front of the tyre with a staggered stance, while gripping the sledge-hammer. Raise the sledgehammer up above the body. Powerfully swing the sledge down to the tyre as hard as you can. As the hammer is lowering your upper hand should slide down to meet the lower hand. Repeat for reps (ensure both sides of the body are trained by switching sides). Notes: Your dominant hand should be higher up the shaft of the sledgehammer, while your non-dominant hand is gripping at the base. Never sacrifice form or control of the hammer and control the impact at all times. Maintain a controlled yet fast and intense pace (don't be tempted by the heaviest sledge in the store). Tip: If you'd like to use your tyre indoors but want to save your floor then place the tyre on top of an old cushion or thick blanket to absorb the impact and prevent friction.

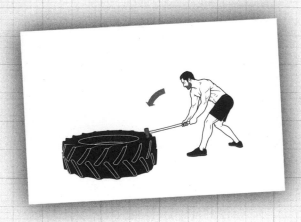

Tyre Flips

Get set on a deep squat, with hips low and pushed back, feet shoulder-width apart. Make sure your knees and feet are aligned. Place hands under the tyre, fingers spread wide. Hips should be pushed back with your head up, shoulders wide. Press your chest against the tyre. Fix arms and shoulders in position, with elbows just slightly flexed. Maintain a flat back and head-up posture as you drive powerfully up through the legs and hips. Generate enough momentum during the initial lift to allow you to get under the tyre, switching from an underhand pull position to a pushing/pressing position using the heel of the hand. Step forward and use your whole body to drive the tyre up and over. Focus on flipping and lifting in one smooth action, working quickly and with good technique.

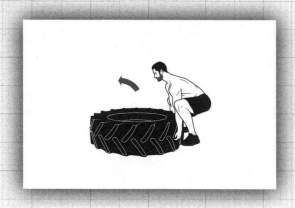

Bear Hug Carry

This involves wrapping your arms around the object (examples include a keg, bumper plate, sandbag or tree) and lifting it to around chest height, holding it securely against your chest. Make sure your fingers are not clasped at the front. The position of the object you are carrying against your chest makes breathing a challenge, which adds to the difficulty of the exercise as a whole.

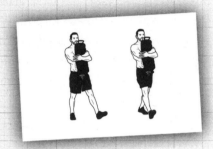

Plate Pinch Farmer's Walk

The plate pinch carry is a variation of the farmer's walk and an exercise used to strengthen the muscles of the forearms. Grasp a plate in each hand using just your fingers. While maintaining an active shoulder position, hold the plates by your side and walk for a designated distance or amount of time (to start, I recommend getting two 10 kg plates, preferably smooth iron plates).

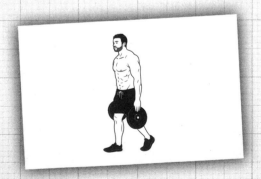

ENDNOTES

PART 1 | WHY WE ADVENTURE

1   Matthews LJ and Butler PM (2011). 'Novelty-seeking DRD4 polymorphisms are associated with human migration distance out-of-Africa after controlling for neutral population gene structure.' *American Journal of Physical Anthropology* **145**(3):382–9.

2   Reinert E, Aslaksen I, Eira I, Mathiesen S, Reinert H and Turi E (2009). 'Adapting to climate change in Sámi reindeer herding: The nation-state as problem and solution.' In: Adger W, Lorenzoni I and O'Brien K (eds) *Adapting to Climate Change: Thresholds, Values, Governance.* Cambridge University Press, Cambridge.

PART 2 | HOW TO ADVENTURE

1   Naclerio F, Moody J and Chapman M (2013). 'Applied periodization: A methodological approach.' *Journal of Human Sport and Exercise* **8**(2):350–66.

2   Pedemonte J (1986). 'Foundations of training periodization Part I: historical outline.' *Strength & Conditioning Journal* **8**(3):62–6.

3   Gamble P (2006). 'Periodization of training for team sports athletes.' *Strength & Conditioning Journal* **28**(5):56–66.

4   Baker D (1998). 'Applying the in-season periodization of strength and power training to football.' *Strength & Conditioning Journal* **20**(2):18–27.

5   Plisk SS and Stone MH (2003). 'Periodization strategies.' *Strength & Conditioning Journal* **25**(6):19–37.

6   Tschiene P (2000). 'Il nuovo orientamento delle structure dell'allenamento.' *Scuola dello Sport* **XIX**:47–8.

7   Verkhoshansky Y (1998). 'Main features of modern scientific sports training theory.' *New Studies in Athletics* **13**(3):9–20.

8 Wathen D, Baechle TR and Earle RW (2008). 'Periodization.' In: Earle RW and Baechle TR (eds) *Essential of Strength Training and Conditioning*. Human Kinetics, Champaign, IL.

9 Turner A (2011). 'The science and practice of periodization: a brief review.' *Strength & Conditioning Journal* **33**(1):34–46.

10 McHugh MP and Tetro DT (2003). 'Changes in the relationship between joint angle and torque production associated with the repeated bout effect.' *Journal of Sports Sciences* **21**(11):927–32.

11 Kiely J (2012). 'Periodization paradigms in the 21st century: evidence-led or tradition-driven?' *International Journal of Sports Physiology and Performance* **7**(3):242–50.

12 This data was collected using the official Olympic.org site, as well as a spreadsheet from the Guardian that includes data from 1896–2008 (available here), 2012 and 2016 data was compared with that from *Encyclopaedia Britannica*, and several news outlets were used to update the table when medals were reassigned (i.e. for doping offences).

13 'Childhood obesity rates rise 10-fold since the '70s', medicalnewstoday.com

14 npr.com

15 Tucker R and Collins M. *What Makes Champions? A Review of The Relative Contribution of Genes and Training to Sporting Success.* Br J Sports Med. 2012 Jun;**46**(8):555–61.

16 'How the body recovers from an ultramarathon: new study reveals keys to recovery after long-distance endurance runs.' AAP Annual Meeting, February 2016. *American Journal of Physical Medicine & Rehabilitation.*

17 Knechtle B and Nikolaidis PT (2018). 'Physiology and pathophysiology in ultra-marathon running.' *Frontiers in Physiology* **9**: 634.

18 Longo A, Siffredi C, Cardey M, Aquilino G and Lentini N (2016). 'Age of peak performance in Olympic sports: a comparative research among disciplines.' *Journal of Human Sport and Exercise* **11**(1): 31–41.

19 Akil H, Young E, Walker JM, and Watson SJ (1986). 'The many possible roles of opioids and related peptides in stress-induced analgesia.' *Annals of the New York Academy of Sciences* **467**:140–53.

20 Butler RK and Finn DP (2009). 'Stress-induced analgesia.' *Progress in Neurobiology* **88**:184–202.

21 Parikh D, Hamid A, Friedman TC, et al. (2011). 'Stress-induced analgesia and endogenous opioid peptides: the importance of stress duration.' *European Journal of Pharmacology* **650**(2-3):563–7.

22 Scott A, Heinlein, PT and Cosgarea AJ (2010). 'Biomechanical considerations in the competitive swimmer's shoulder.' *Sports Health* **2**(6): 519–25.

23 Smidt N, De Vet HC, Bouter LM, et al. (2005). 'Effectiveness of exercise therapy: a best-evidence summary of systematic reviews.' *Australian Journal of Physiotherapy* **51**:71–85.

24 Taylor NF, Dodd KJ and Damiano DL (2005). 'Progressive resistance exercise in physical therapy: a summary of systematic reviews.' *Physical Therapist* **85**:1208–23.

25 Khan KM and Mechanotherapy SA (2009). 'How physical therapists' prescription of exercise promotes tissue repair.' *British Journal of Sports Medicine* **43**(4):247–52.

26 Duncan RL and Turner CH (1995). 'Mechanotransduction and the functional response of bone to mechanical strain.' *Calcified Tissue International* **57**(5):344–58.

27 McElhaney JH, Stalnaker R and Bullard R (1968). 'Electric fields and bone loss of disuse.' *Journal of Biomechanics* **1**(1):47–52.

28 Bompa T (1999). *Periodization: Theory and Methodology of Training (4th edition)*. Human Kinetics, Champaign, IL.

29 Lauersen JB, Bertelsen DM and Andersen LB (2014). 'The effectiveness of exercise interventions to prevent sports injuries: a systematic review and meta-analysis of randomised controlled trials.' *British Journal of Sports Medicine* **48**(11):871–7.

30 Lauersen JB, Andersen TE and Andersen LB (2018). 'Strength training as superior, dose-dependent and safe prevention of acute and overuse sports injuries: a systematic review, qualitative analysis and meta-analysis.' *British Journal of Sports Medicine* **52**(24): 1557–63.

31 Askling C, Karlsson J and Thorstensson A (2003). 'Hamstring injury occurrence in elite soccer players after preseason strength training with eccentric overload.' *Scandinavian Journal of Medicine and Science in Sports* **13**(4):244–50.

32 Hejna WF, Rosenberg A, Buturusis DJ and Krieger A (1982). 'The prevention of sports injuries in high school students through strength training.' *Strength & Conditioning Journal* **4**(1):28–31.

33 Skelton DA and Beyer N (2003). 'Exercise and injury prevention in older people.' *Scandinavian Journal of Medicine and Science in Sports* **13**(1):77–85.

34 Cools AM, Witvrouw EE, Declercq GA, et al. (2004). 'Evaluation of isokinetic force production and associated muscle activity in the scapular rotators during a protraction–retraction movement in overhead athletes with impingement symptoms.' *British Journal of Sports Medicine* **38**:64–8.

35 Kelley MJ (1995). 'Anatomic and biomechanical rationale for rehabilitation of the athlete's shoulder.' *Journal of Sport Rehabilitation* **4**(2):122–54.

36 Treiber FA, et al. (1998). 'Effects of Theraband and lightweight dumbbell training on shoulder rotation torque and serve performance in college tennis players.' *American Journal of Sports Medicine* **26**(4):510–15.

37 Page PA, Lamberth J, Abadie B, Boling R, Collins R and Linton R (1993). 'Posterior rotator cuff strengthening using Theraband® in a functional diagonal pattern in collegiate baseball pitchers.' *Journal of Athletic Training* **28**(4):346–54.

38 Washburn S (1971). 'The study of human evolution.' In: Dolhinow P and Sarich V (eds) *Background for Man: Readings in Physical Anthropology.* Little Brown and Co., Boston, MA.

39 Chang Y-H, Bertram JEA and Lee DV (2000). 'External forces and torques generated by the brachiating white-handed gibbon (Hylobates Lar).' *American Journal of Physical Anthropology* **113**: 201–16.

40 Pennock ET (2013). 'From gibbons to gymnasts: a look at the biomechanics and neurophysiology of brachiation in gibbons and its human rediscovery.' *Student Works 2.*

41 Bertram JEA (2004). 'New perspectives on brachiation mechanics.' *American Journal of Physical Anthropology* **47**:100–17.

42 Blue RS, Bayuse TM, Daniels VR, Wotring VE, Rahul S, Mulcahy RA and Antonsen EL (2019). 'Supplying a pharmacy for NASA exploration spaceflight: challenges and current understanding.' *NPJ Microgravity* **5**:14.

43 Arnauld E, Nicogossian RB and House NG (2017). 'In-flight medical monitoring, space biology and medicine.' In: *Health, Performance, and Safety of Space Crews Volume IV.* Chap. 4.

44 Bacon D, Butler I, Fotedar L, Jaweed M, Leblanc A, Narayana P, Schneider V and Slopis J (1992). 'Magnetic resonance imaging (MRI) of skeletal muscles in astronauts after 9 days of space flight.' *Aerospace Medical Association*. Aerospace Medical Association 63rd Annual Scientific Meeting Program.

45 Ireland A, Maden-Wilkinson T, McPhee J, Cooke K, Narici M, Degens H and Rittweger J (2013). 'Upper limb muscle–bone asymmetries and bone adaptation in elite youth tennis players.' *Medicine & Science in Sports & Exercise* 45(9):1749–58.

46 Kannus P, Haapasalo H, Sankelo M, Sievänen H, Pasanen M, Heinonen A, Oja P and Vuori I (1995). 'Effect of starting age of physical activity on bone mass in the dominant arm of tennis and squash players.' *Annals of International Medicine* 123:27–31.

47 Franettovich M, Hides J, Mendis MD, et al. (2011). 'Muscle imbalance among elite athletes.' *British Journal of Sports Medicine* 45:348–49.

48 Grimm D, Grosse J, Wehland M, Mann V, Reseland JE, Alamelu S and Corydon TJ (2016). 'The impact of microgravity on bone in humans.' *Bone* 87:44–56.

49 Derendorf H (2013). 'Pharmacokinetic/pharmacodynamic consequences of space flight.' *Journal of Clinical Pharmacology* 34(6): 684–91.

50 Wall BT, Dirks ML and Van Loon LJ (2013) 'Skeletal muscle atrophy during short-term disuse: implications for age-related sarcopenia.' *Ageing Research Reviews* 12(4):898–906.

51 Haff G (2013). 'Periodization of training.' In: Chandler TJ and Brown LE (eds) *Conditioning for Strength and Human Performance*. Lippincott Williams & Wilkins, PA.

52 Friden J and Lieber RL (1992). 'Structural and mechanical basis of exercise-induced muscle injury.' *Medicine and Science in Sports and Exercise* 24(5):521–30.

53 Bompa T (1993). *Periodization of Strength: The New Wave in Strength Training*. Veritas, Toronto.

54 Taunton JE, Ryan MB, Clement DB, McKenzie DC, Lloyd-Smith DR and Zumbo BD (2003). 'A prospective study of running injuries: the Vancouver Sun Run "in training" clinics.' *British Journal of Sports Medicine* 37:239–44.

55 Van Mechelen W (1992). 'Running injuries, a review of the epidemiological literature.' *Sports Medicine* 14(5):320–35.

56 Van Gent RM, Siem D, Van Middlekoop M, Van Os AG, Bierma-Zein-stra AMA and Koes BW (2007). 'Incidence and determinants of lower extremity running injuries in long distance runners: a systematic review.' *British Journal of Sports Medicine* **41**:469–807.

57 Nesse RM and Williams GC (1994). *Why We Get Sick: The New Science of Darwinian Medicine*. Vantage, NY.

58 Davis IS (2014). 'The re-emergence of the minimal running shoe.' *Journal of Orthopaedic & Sports Physical Therapy* **44**(10):775–84.

59 Lieberman DE (2012). 'What we can learn about running from barefoot running: an evolutionary medical perspective.' *Exercise and Sport Sciences Reviews* **40**(2):63–72.

60 McKeon PO, Hertel J, Bramble D, et al. (2015). 'The foot core system: a new paradigm for understanding intrinsic foot muscle function.' *British Journal of Sports Medicine* **49**(5):290.

61 Venkadesan M, Yawar A, Eng CM, et al. (1991). 'Stiffness of the human foot and evolution of the transverse arch.' *Nature* **579**:97–100.

62 Alexander RM (1991). 'Energy-saving mechanisms in walking and running.' *Journal of Experimental Biology* **160**:55–69.

63 Lieberman DE (2014). *The Story of the Human Body: Evolution, Health, and Disease*. Allen Lane, London.

64 Perl DP, Daoud AI and Lieberman DE (2012). 'Effects of footwear and strike type on running economy.' *Medicine and Science in Sports and Exercise* **44**(7):1335–43.

65 Lieberman DE (2012). 'What we can learn about running from barefoot running: an evolutionary medical perspective.' *Exercises and Sport Sciences Review* **40**(2):63–72.

66 Hasegawa H, Yamauchi T and Kraemer WJ (2007). 'Foot strike patterns of runners at the 15-km point during an elite-level half marathon.' *Journal of Strength and Conditioning Research* **21**(3):888–93.

67 Francis P, Oddy C and Johnson MI (2017). 'Reduction in plantar heel pain and a return to sport after a barefoot running intervention in a female triathlete with plantar fasciitis.' *International Journal of Athletic Therapy & Training* **22**(5):26–32.

68 Pohl MB, Hamill J and Davis IS (2009). 'Biomechanical and anatomic factors associated with a history of plantar fasciitis in female runners.' *Clinical Journal of Sport Medicine* **19**(5):372–6.

69 Daoud AI, Geissler GJ, Wang F, et al. (2012). 'Foot strike and injury rates in endurance runners: a retrospective study.' *Medicine and Science in Sports and Exercise* **44**(7):1325–34.

70 Daoud AI, Geissler GJ, Wang F, et al. (2012). 'Foot strike and injury rates in endurance runners: a retrospective study.' *Medicine and Science in Sports and Exercise* **44**(7):1325–34.

71 Francis P and Schofield G (2020). 'From barefoot hunter gathering to shod pavement pounding. Where to from here? A narrative review.' *BMJ Open Sport and Exercise Medicine* **6**.

72 Warne JP and Gruber AH (2017). 'Transitioning to minimal footwear: a systematic review of methods and future clinical recommendations.' *Sports Medicine Open* **3**(1):33.

73 Kreher JB (2016). 'Diagnosis and prevention of overtraining syndrome: an opinion on education strategies.' *Journal of Sports Medicine* **7**:115–22.

74 Halson SL and Jeukendrup AE (2004). 'Does overtraining exist? An analysis of overreaching and overtraining research.' *Sports Medicine* **34**(14):967–81.

75 Gouarné C, Groussard C, Gratas-Delamarche A, Delamarche P and Duclos M (2005). 'Overnight urinary cortisol and cortisone add new insights into adaptation to training.' *Medicine and Science in Sports and Exercise* **37**(7):1157–67.

76 Pichot V, Roche F and Gaspoz JM (2000). 'Relation between heart rate variability and training load in middle-distance runners.' *Medicine and Science in Sports and Exercise* **32**(10):1729–36.

77 Koutedakis Y (2000). '"Burnout" in dance: the physiological viewpoint.' *Journal of Dance Medicine & Science* **4**(4):122–7.

78 Parker S, Brukner P and Rosier M (1996). 'Chronic fatigue syndrome and the athlete.' *Sports Medicine, Training and Rehabilitation* **6**(4):269–78.

79 Lehmann MJ, Lormes W, Opitz-Gress A, Steinacker JM, Netzer N, Foster C and Gastmann U (1997). 'Training and overtraining: an overview and experimental results in endurance sports.' *Journal of Sports Medicine and Physical Fitness* **37**(1):7–17.

80 McLay RN, Klam WP and Volkert SL (2010). 'Insomnia is the most commonly reported symptom and predicts other symptoms of post-traumatic stress disorder in US service members returning from military deployments.' *Military Medicine* **175**(10):759–62.

81 Kujawski S, et al. (2018). 'The impact of total sleep deprivation upon cognitive functioning in firefighters.' *Neuropsychiatric Disease and Treatment* **14**:1171–81.

82 Good CH, Brager AJ, Capaldi VF and Mysliwiec V (2020). 'Sleep in the United States military.' *Neuropsychopharmacology* **45**(1):176–91.

83 Peterson AL, Goodie JL, Satterfield WA and Brim WL (2008). 'Sleep disturbance during military deployment.' *Military Medicine* **173**(3):230–5.

84 Bramoweth AD and Germain A (2013). 'Deployment-related insomnia in military personnel and veterans.' *Current Psychiatry Reports* **15**(10):401.

85 Shapiro CM, Bortz R, Mitchell D, Bartel P and Jooste P (1981). 'Slow-wave sleep: a recovery period after exercise.' *Science* **214**(4526):1253–4.

86 Aristotle (2014). *On Sleep and Sleeplessness*. Beare JI (trans.). Kindle Edition.

87 Dijk DJ and Czeisler CA (1995). 'Contribution of the circadian pacemaker and the sleep homeostat to sleep propensity, sleep structure, electroencephalographic slow waves, and sleep spindle activity in humans.' *Journal of Neuroscience* **15**(5):3526–38.

88 Reppert SM and Weaver DR (2002). 'Coordination of circadian timing in mammals.' *Nature* **418**(6901):935–41

89 Arendt J and Broadway J (1997). 'Light and melatonin as zeitgebers in man.' *Journal of Biological and Medical Rhythm Research* **4**(2):273–82.

90 Smolensky MH and Haus E (2001). 'Circadian rhythms and clinical medicine with applications to hypertension.' *American Journal of Hypertension* **14**(S6):280S–290S.

91 Lieberman HR, Tharion WJ, Shukitt-Hale B, et al. (2002). 'Effects of caffeine, sleep loss, and stress on cognitive performance and mood during U.S. Navy SEAL training.' *Psychopharmacology* **164**(3):250–61.

92 Tharion WJ, Shukitt-Hale B and Lieberman HR (2003). 'Caffeine effects on marksmanship during high-stress military training with 72 hour sleep deprivation.' *Aviation, Space and Environmental Medicine* **74**(4):309–14.

93 Goldstein A, Warren R and Kaizer S (1965). 'Psychotropic effects of caffeine in man. I. Individual differences in sensitivity to caffeine-induced wakefulness.' *Journal of Pharmacology and Experimental Therapeutics* **149**:156–59.

94 Weiss B and Laties VG (1962). 'Enhancement of human performance by caffeine and the amphetamines.' *Pharmacological Reviews* **14**:1–36.

95 Penetar D, McCann U, Thorne D, et al. (1993). 'Caffeine reversal of sleep deprivation effects on alertness and mood.' *Psychopharmacology* **112**(2-3):359–65.

96 Graham TE (2001). 'Caffeine and Exercise.' *Sports Medicine* **31**(11):785–807.

97 Ivy J, Kammer L, Ding Z, Wang B, Bernard J, Liao Y-H and Hwang J-Y. (2009). 'Improved cycling time-trial performance after ingestion of a caffeine energy drink.' *International Journal of Sport Nutrition and Exercise Metabolism* **19**(1):61–78.

98 Stuart G, Hopkins W; Cook C and Cairns S (2005). 'Multiple effects of caffeine on simulated high-intensity team-sport performance.' *Medicine and Science in Sports and Exercise* **37**(11):1998–2005.

99 Berglund B and Hemmingsson P (1982). 'Effects of caffeine ingestion on exercise performance at low and high altitudes in cross-country skiers.' *International Journal of Sports Medicine* **3**(4):234–6.

100 Essig D, Costili DL and Van Handel PJ (1980). 'Effects of caffeine ingestion on utilization of muscle glycogen and lipid during leg ergometer cycling.' *International Journal of Sports Medicine* **1**:86–90.

101 Lopes JM, Aubier M, Jardim J, Aranda JV and Macklem PT (1983). 'Effect of caffeine on skeletal muscle function before and after fatigue.' *Journal of Applied Physiology* **54**(5):1303–5.

102 Sinclair CJD and Geiger J (2000). 'Caffeine use in sports. a pharmacological review.' *Journal of Sports Medicine and Physical Fitness* **40**(1):71–9.

103 Lane SC, Areta JL, Bird SR, Coffey VG, Burke LM, Desbrow B, Karagounis LG and Hawley JA (2013). 'Caffeine ingestion and cycling power output in a low or normal muscle glycogen state.' *Medicine and Science in Sports and Exercise* **45**(8):1577–84.

104 Graham TE (2001). 'Caffeine and exercise: metabolism, endurance and performance.' *Sports Medicine* **31**(11):785–807.

105 Baratloo A, Rouhipour A, Forouzanfar MM, Safari S, Amiri M and Negida A (2016). 'The role of caffeine in pain management: a brief literature review.' *Anesthesiology and Pain Medicine* **6**(3):e33193.

106 Astorino TA, Terzi MN, Roberson DW, and Burnett TR (2011). 'Effect of caffeine intake on pain perception during high intensity exercise.' *International Journal of Sport Nutrition and Exercise Metabolism* **21**(1):27–32.

107 Duncan M, Stanley M, Parkhouse N, Cook K and Smith M (2011). 'Acute caffeine ingestion enhances strength performance and reduces perceived exertion and muscle pain perception during resistance exercise.' *European Journal of Sport Science* **15**:1–8.

108 Motl RW, O'Connor PJ and Dishman RK (2003). 'Effect of caffeine on perceptions of leg muscle pain during moderate intensity cycling exercise.' *Journal of Pain* **4**(6):316–21.

109 Derry CJ, Derry S and Moore RA (2012).' Caffeine as an analgesic adjuvant for acute pain in adults.' *Cochrane Database of Systematic Reviews* **3**:CD009281.

110 Rechtschaffen A (1998). 'Current perspectives on the function of sleep.' *Perspectives in Biology and Medicine* **41**(3):359–90.

111 Assefa SZ, Diaz-Abad M, Wickwire EM and Scharf SM (2015). 'The functions of sleep.' *AIMS Neuroscience* **2**(3):155–71.

112 Kovalzon VM (2009). 'Some notes on the biography of Maria Manasseina.' *Journal of the History of the Neurosciences* **18**(3):312–19.

113 Bentivoglio M and Grassi-Zucconi G (1997). 'The pioneering experimental studies on sleep deprivation.' *Sleep* **20**(7):570–6.

114 West LJ, Janszen HH, Lester BK and Cornelisoon FS (1962). 'The psychosis of sleep deprivation.' *Some Biological Aspects of Schizophrenic Behaviour* **96**(1):66–70.

115 Hurdiel R, Pezé T, Daugherty J, Girard J, Poussel M, Poletti L, Basset P and Theunynck D (2015). 'Combined effects of sleep deprivation and strenuous exercise on cognitive performances during The North Face® Ultra Trail du Mont Blanc® (UTMB®).' *Journal of Sports Sciences* **33**(7):670–4.

116 Babkoff H, Sing HC, Thorne DR, Genser SG and Hegge FW (1989). 'Perceptual distortions and hallucinations reported during the course of sleep deprivation.' *Perceptual and Motor Skills* **68**(3): 787–98.

117 Chrousos G, Vgontzas AN and Kritikou I (2016). 'HPA axis and sleep.' In: Feingold KR, Anawalt B, Boyce A, et al. (eds), Endotext [Internet], South Dartmouth, MA. https://www.ncbi.nlm.nih.gov/books/NBK279071/.

118 Takahashi Y, Kipnis DM and Daughaday WH (1968). 'Growth hormone secretion during sleep.' *Journal of Clinical Investigation* **47**(9):2079–90.

119 Brand S, Beck J, Gerber M, Hatzinger M and Holsboer-Trachsler E (2010). 'Evidence of favorable sleep-EEG patterns in adolescent male vigorous football players compared to controls.' *World Journal of Biological Psychiatry* **11**(2-2):465–75.

120 Mah CD, Mah KE, Kezirian EJ and Dement WC (2011). 'The effects of sleep extension on the athletic performance of collegiate basketball players.' *Sleep* **34**(7):943–50.

121 Diekelmann S (2014). 'Sleep for cognitive enhancement.' *Frontiers in Systems Neuroscience* **8**(46). https://doi.org/10.3389/fnsys.

122 Pilcher JJ and Huffcutt AI (1996). 'Effects of sleep deprivation on performance: a meta-analysis.' *Sleep* **19**(4):318-26.

123 Honn KA, Hinson JM, Whitney P and Van Dongen HPA (2019). 'Cognitive flexibility: a distinct element of performance impairment due to sleep deprivation.' *Accident Analysis & Prevention* **126**:191-7.

124 Alhola P and Polo-Kantola P (2007). 'Sleep deprivation: impact on cognitive performance.' *Neuropsychiatric Disease and Treatment* **3**(5):553-67.

125 Van Dongen HPA, Maislin G, Mullington JM and Dinges DF (2003). 'The cumulative cost of additional wakefulness: dose–response effects on neurobehavioral functions and sleep physiology from chronic sleep restriction and total sleep deprivation.' *Sleep* **26**(2):117-26.

126 Luckhaupt S (2012). 'Short sleep duration among workers – United States, 2010.' *Morbidity and Mortality Weekly Report* **61**:281-5.

127 Watson NF, Badr MS, Belenky G, et al. (2015). 'Joint consensus statement of the American Academy of Sleep Medicine and Sleep Research Society on the recommended amount of sleep for a healthy adult: methodology and discussion.' *Sleep* **38**(8):1161-83.

128 Richards A, Inslicht SS, Metzler TJ, Mohlenhoff BS, Rao MN, O'Donovan A and Neylan TC (2017). 'Sleep and cognitive performance from teens to old age: more is not better.' *Sleep* **40**(1):zsw029. doi: 10.1093/sleep/zsw029.

129 Shochat T, Cohen-Zion M and Tzischinsky O (2014). 'Functional consequences of inadequate sleep in adolescents: a systematic review.' *Sleep Medicine Reviews* **18**(1):75-87.

130 Ohayon MM, Carskadon MA, Guilleminault C and Vitiello MV (2004). 'Meta-analysis of quantitative sleep parameters from childhood to old age in healthy individuals: developing normative sleep values across the human lifespan.' *Sleep* **27**(7):1255-73.

131 Beccuti G and Pannain S (2011). 'Sleep and obesity.' *Current Opinion in Clinical Nutrition and Metabolic Care* **14**(4):402-12.

132 Al-Abri MA, et al. (2016). 'Habitual sleep deprivation is associated with type 2 diabetes: a case-control study.' *Oman Medical Journal* **31**(6):399-403.

133 Nagai M, et al (2010). 'Sleep duration as a risk factor for cardiovascular disease: a review of the recent literature.' *Current Cardiology Reviews* **6**(1):54-61.

134 Owens J (2014). 'Insufficient sleep in adolescents and young adults: an update on causes and consequences.' *Pediatrics* **134**(3): e921–e932.

135 Chattu VK, Manzar MD, Kumary S, Burman D, Spence DW and Pandi-Perumal SR (2018). 'The global problem of insufficient sleep and its serious public health implications.' *Healthcare* **7**(1):1.

136 Selmaoui B and Touitou Y (2003). 'Reproducibility of the circadian rhythms of serum cortisol and melatonin in healthy subjects: a study of three different 24-h cycles over six weeks.' *Life Sciences* **73**(26): 3339–49.

137 Wright, KP Jr, et al. (2013). 'Entrainment of the human circadian clock to the natural light–dark cycle.' *Current Biology* **23**(16): 1554–8.

138 Chaudhary NS, Grandner MA, Jackson NJ and Chakravorty S (2016). 'Caffeine consumption, insomnia, and sleep duration: results from a nationally representative sample.' *Nutrition* **32**(11-12):1193–9.

139 Roehrs T, et al. (2008). 'Caffeine: sleep and daytime sleepiness.' *Sleep Medicine Reviews* **12**(2):153–62.

140 Shilo L, Sabbah H, Hadari R, et al. (2002). 'The effects of coffee consumption on sleep and melatonin secretion.' *Sleep Medicine* **3**(3):271–3.

141 Clark I and Landolt HP (2016). 'Coffee, caffeine, and sleep.' *Sleep Medicine Reviews* **31**:70–8.

142 Drake C, Roehrs T, Shambroom J and Roth T (2013). 'Caffeine effects on sleep taken 0, 3, or 6 hours before going to bed.' *Journal of Clinical Sleep Medicine* **9**(11):1195–1200.

143 Vanderlinden J, Boen F and Van Uffelen JGZ (2020). 'Effects of physical activity programs on sleep outcomes in older adults: a systematic review.' *International Journal of Behavioural Nutrition and Physical Activity* **17**(11):1–15.

144 Dworak M, Diel P, Voss S, Hollmann W and Strüder HK (2007). 'Intense exercise increases adenosine concentrations in rat brain: implications for a homeostatic sleep drive.' *Neuroscience* **150**(4):789–95.

145 Brupbacher G, Gerger H, Wechsler M, et al. (2019). 'The effects of aerobic, resistance, and meditative movement exercise on sleep in individuals with depression: protocol for a systematic review and network meta-analysis.' *Systematic Reviews* **8**(105).

146 D'Aurea C, Poyares D, Passos G, Santana M, Youngstedt S, Lino de Souza A, Bicudo J, Tufik S and De Mello M (2018). 'Effects of resist-

ance exercise training and stretching on chronic insomnia.' *Brazilian Journal of Psychiatry* **41**(1):51–7.

147 Okamoto-Mizuno K and Mizuno K (2012). 'Effects of thermal environment on sleep and circadian rhythm.' *Journal of Physiological Anthropology* **31**(1):14.

148 Obradovich N, et al. (2017). 'Nighttime temperature and human sleep loss in a changing climate.' *Science Advances* **3**(5):e1601555.

149 Howatson G, Bell PG, Tallent J, et al. (2012). 'Effect of tart cherry juice (Prunus cerasus) on melatonin levels and enhanced sleep quality.' *European Journal of Nutrition* **51**(8):909–16.

150 Folland JP, Irish CS, Roberts JC, Tarr JE and Jones DA (2002). 'Fatigue is not a necessary stimulus for strength gains during resistance training.' *British Journal of Sports Medicine* **36**(5):370–4.

151 Sampson JA and Groeller H (2016). 'Is repetition failure critical for the development of muscle hypertrophy and strength?' *Scandinavian Journal of Medicine & Science in Sports* **26**(4):375–83.

152 Ho R (1987). 'Talent identification in China.' In: Petiot B, Salmela JH and Hoshizaki TB (eds), *World Identification for Gymnastic Talent*. Sports Psyche Editions, Montreal.

153 Hartley G (1988). 'A comparative view of talent selection for sport in two socialist states – the USSR and the GDR – with particular reference to gymnastics.' In: *The Growing Child in Competitive Sport*. The National Coaching Foundation, Leeds.

154 Bompa TO (1985). 'Talent identification.' In: *Sports: Science Periodical on Research and Technology in Sport, Physical Testing, GN-1*. Coaching Association of Canada, Ottawa.

155 Lawrence SV (1992). 'China's sporting dreams.' *U.S. News and World Report* **112**:59.

156 Dvorkin LS (1992). *Weightlifting and Age (Scientific and Pedagogical Fundamentals of a Multi-Year System of Training Junior Weightlifters*. Charniga A (trans.). Sportivny Press, Livonia, MI.

157 Drabik J. (1996). *Children and Sports Training: How Your Future Champions Should Exercise to be Healthy, Fit, and Happy*. Kurtz T (trans.). Stadion Publishing Company Inc., Island Pond, VT.

158 Smoll FL and Smith RE (2002). *Children and Youth in Sport: A Biopsychosocial Perspective (2nd Edition)*. Kendall/Hunt, Dubuque, IA.

159 Ozolin NG (1949). *Fundamentals of Special Strength-Training in Sport*. Charniga A (trans.). Sportivny Press, Livonia, MI.

160 Kurtz T (2001). *Science of Sports Training: How to Plan and Control for Peak Performance (2nd Edition)*. Stadion Publishing Company Inc., Island Pond, VT.

161 Harre D (1982). 'Trainingslehre.' In: Bompa TO (2000). *Total Training for Young Children*. Human Kinetics, Champaign, IL.

162 Nagorni MF (1978). 'Facts and fiction regarding junior's training.' In: Bompa TO (2000). *Total Training for Young Children*. Human Kinetics, Champaign, IL.

163 Myslinski T (2005). *The Development of the Russian Conjugate Sequence System*. Zugriff unter http://www.elitefts.com/documents/TomMyslinski.pdf.

164 Wathen D and Baechle T (2008). *'Periodization' Essentials of Strength Training and Conditioning (3rd Edition)*. Human Kinetics/National Strength & Conditioning Association.

165 Medvedyev AS (1989). *A System of Multi-Year Training in Weightlifting*. Charniga A (trans.). Sportivny Press, Livonia, MI.

166 Tipton MJ, Collier N, Corbett J, Massey H and Harper M (2017). 'Cold water immersion: kill or cure?' *Experimental Physiology* **102**(11):1335–55.

167 Tipton MJ (2013). 'Sudden cardiac death during open water swimming.' *British Journal of Sports Medicine* **48**(15):1134–5.

168 Bierens JJ, Lunetta P, Tipton MJ and Warner DS (2016). 'Physiology of drowning: a review.' *Physiology (Bethesda)* **31**(2):147–66.

169 Gilbert N (2016). 'Green space: a natural high.' *Nature* **531**(7594): S56–7.

170 Romet TT (1988). 'Mechanism of after drop after cold water immersion.' *Journal of Applied Physiology* **65**(4):1535–8.

171 Giesbrecht GG and Hayward JS (2006). 'Problems and complications with cold-water rescue.' *Wilderness & Environmental Medicine* **17**(1): 26–30.

172 Golden F and Tipton MJ (2002). *Essentials of Sea Survival*. Human Kinetics, Champaign, IL.

173 Nuckton TJ, Claman DM, Goldreich D, Wendt FC and Nuckton JG (2000). 'Hypothermia and afterdrop following open water swimming: the Alcatraz/San Francisco swim study.' *American Journal of Emergency Medicine* **18**(6):703–7.

174 Thompson RF and Spencer WA (1996). 'Habituation: A model phenomenon for the study of neuronal substrates of behaviour.' *Psychological Review* **73**(1):16–43.

175 Van Paridon KN, Timmis MA, Nevison CM and Bristow M (2017). 'The anticipatory stress response to sport competition: a systematic review with meta-analysis of cortisol reactivity.' *BMJ Open Sport & Exercise Medicine* **3**(1):e000261.

176 Vera FM, Manzaneque JM, Carranque GA, Rodríguez-Peña FM, Sánchez-Montes S and Blanca MJ (2018). 'Endocrine modulation in long-term karate practitioners.' *Evidence-Based Complementary and Alternative Medicine* Article ID 1654148.

177 Salvador A (2005). 'Coping with competitive situations in humans.' *Neuroscience & Bio-behavioral Reviews* **29**(1):195–205.

178 Meyer VJ, Lee Y, Böttger C, Leonbacher U, Allison AL and Shirtcliff EA (2015). 'Experience, cortisol reactivity, and the coordination of emotional responses to skydiving.' *Frontiers of Human Neuroscience* **25**(9):138.

179 Burstein R, Coward AW, Askew WE, Carmel K, Irving C, Shpilberg O, Moran D, Pikarsky A, Ginot G, Sawyer M, Golan R and Epstein Y (1996). 'Energy expenditure variations in soldiers performing military activities under cold and hot climate conditions.' *Military Medicine* **161**(12):750–4.

180 Andersen KL, Loyning Y, Nelms JD, Wilson O, Fox RH and Bolstad A (1960). 'Metabolic and thermal response to a moderate cold exposure in nomadic Lapps.' *Journal of Applied Physiology* **15**(4):649–53.

181 Wesołowski R, Mila-Kierzkowska CA, Woźniak A, Buraczynski T and Sutkowy P (2013). 'Body composition analysis in regular winter swimmers and people who do not use this form of recreation.' *Medical and Biological Sciences* **27**:47–52.

182 Griggio MA (1998). 'Thermogenic mechanisms in cold-acclimated animals.' *Brazilian Journal of Medical and Biological Research* **21**(2): 171–6.

183 Periasamy M, Herrera JL and Reis F (2017). 'Skeletal muscle thermogenesis and its role in whole body energy metabolism.' *Diabetes & Metabolism Journal* **41**(5):327–36.

184 Nepos C (2017). *Complete Works of Cornelius Nepos (Illustrated)*. Delphi Classics.

185 Midgley AW, McNaughton LR and Jones AM (2007). 'Training to enhance the physiological determinants of long-distance running performance: can valid recommendations be given to runners and coaches based on current scientific knowledge?' *Sports Medicine* **37**(10):857–80.

186 Withers RT, Sherman WM and Miller JM (1981). 'Specificity of the anaerobic threshold in endurance trained cyclists and runners.' *European Journal of Applied Physiology* 47(1):93–104.

187 Ghosh AK (2004). 'Anaerobic threshold: its concept and role in endurance sport.' *Malaysian Journal of Medical Sciences* 11(1):24–36.

188 Rost R (1997). 'The athlete's heart. Historical perspectives – solved and unsolved problems.' *Cardiology Clinics* 15(3):493–512.

189 Abergel E, Chatellier G, Hagege AA, et al. (2004). 'Serial left ventricular adaptations in world-class professional cyclists: implications for disease screening and follow-up.' *Journal of the American College of Cardiology* 44(1):144–9.

190 Arbab-Zadeh A, Perhonen M, Howden E, et al. (2014). 'Cardiac remodeling in response to 1 year of intensive endurance training.' *Circulation* 130(24):2152–61.

191 Blomqvist CG and Saltin B (1983). 'Cardiovascular adaptations to physical training.' *Annual Review of Physiology* 45:169–89.

192 Menshikova EV, Ritov VB, Fairfull L, Ferrell RE, Kelley DE and Goodpaster BH (2006). 'Effects of exercise on mitochondrial content and function in aging human skeletal muscle.' *Journals of Gerontology Series A* 61(6):534–40.

193 Convertino VF (1991). 'Blood volume: its adaptation to endurance training.' *Medicine and Science in Sports and Exercise* 23(12):1338–48.

194 Goodman JM, Liu, PP and Green HJ (2005). 'Left ventricular adaptations following short-term endurance training.' *Journal of Applied Physiology* 98(2):454–60.

195 Goldsmith RL, Bigger JT, Steinman RC and Fleiss JL (1992). 'Comparison of 24-hour parasympathetic activity in endurance-trained and untrained young men.' *Journal of the American College of Cardiology* 20(3):552–8.

196 Epstein Y, Rosenblum J, Burstein R and Sawka MN (1988). 'External load can alter the energy cost of prolonged exercise.' *European Journal of Applied Physiology and Occupational Physiology* 57(2):243–7.

197 Iampietro PF, Vaughan JA, Goldman RF, Kreider MB, Masucci F and Bass DE (1960). 'Heat production from shivering.' *Journal of Applied Physiology* 15(4):632–4.

198 Celi FS, et al. (2010). 'Minimal changes in environmental temperature result in a significant increase in energy expenditure and

changes in the hormonal homeostasis in healthy adults.' *European Journal of Endocrinology* **163**(6):863–72.

199 Van Marken Lichtenbelt WD, Vanhommerig JW, Smulders NM, Drossaerts JMAFL, Kemerink GJ, Bouvy ND, Schrauwen P and Teule GJJ (2009). 'Cold-activated brown adipose tissue in healthy men.' *New England Journal of Medicine* **360**(15):1500–8.

200 Van Marken Lichtenbelt WD, Schrauwen P, Van de Kerckhove S and Westerterp-Plantenga MS (2002). 'Individual variation in body temperature and energy expenditure in response to mild cold.' *American Journal of Physiology-Endocrinology and Metabolism* **282**(5):E1077–83.

201 Clarkson J (2010). *Soup: A Global History.* Reaktion Books, London.

202 Aristotle (1944). *Aristotle in 23 Volumes: Volume 21.* Rackham H (trans.). William Heinemann, London.

203 Cornell T (2002). *War and Games.* Boydell & Brewer, Suffolk.

204 García-Pallarés J and Izquierdo M (2011). 'Strategies to optimize concurrent training of strength and aerobic fitness for rowing and canoeing.' *Sports Medicine* **41**(4):329–43.

205 Reid HL (2012). 'The political heritage of the Olympic Games: relevance, risks, and possible rewards.' *Sport, Ethics and Philosophy* **6**(2):108–22.

206 Fernandez E and Turk DC (1989). 'The utility of cognitive coping strategies for altering pain perception: a meta-analysis.' *Pain* **38**(2):123–35.

207 Egan S (1987). 'Acute-pain tolerance among athletes.' *Canadian Journal of Sport Sciences* **12**(4):175–8.

208 Ryan ED and Kovacic CR (1966). 'Pain tolerance and sports participation.' *Perceptual and Motor Skills* **22**:383–90.

209 Azevedo DC and Samulski DM (2003). 'Assessment of psychological pain management techniques: a comparative study between athletes and non-athletes.' *Revista Brasileira de Medicina do Esporte* **9**(4): 214–22.

210 Leznicka K, Pawlak M, Bialecka M, Safranow K, Spieszny M, Klocek, Tomasz and Cieszczyk P (2016). 'Evaluation of the pain threshold and tolerance of pain by martial arts athletes and non-athletes using a different methods and tools.' *Archives of Budo* **12**:239–45.

211 Jarvis JA (1902). *The Art of Swimming with Notes on Polo and Aids to Life Saving.* Clarke, WH (ed.). Hutchinson, London.

212 Osmond G (2019). 'Swimming instruction trust of America: the Cavill family, borderlands and decentring Australia sport history.' *Sport in History* **39**(1):24–44.

213 Deschodt VJ, Arsac LM and Rouard AH (1999). 'Relative contribution of arms and legs in humans to propulsion in 25-m sprint front-crawl swimming.' *European Journal of Applied Physiology* **80** (3):192–9.

214 Counsilman JE (1968). *The Science of Swimming*. Prentice-Hall, Englewood Cliffs, NJ.

215 Hay JG (1993). *The Biomechanics of Sports Techniques* (4th edition). Prentice Hall, Englewood Cliffs, NJ.

216 Czabanski B and Koszcyc T (1979). 'Relationship of stroke asymmetry and speed of breaststroke swimming.' In: Terauds J and Bedingfield EW (eds.). *Swimming III*. University Park Press, Baltimore, MD.

217 Strzala M, Stanula A, Głab G, et al. (2015). 'Shaping physiological indices, swimming technique, and their influence on 200m breaststroke race in young swimmers.' *Journal of Sports Science and Medicine* **14**(1):110–17.

218 Lätt E, Jürimäe J, Mäestu J, et al. (2010). 'Physiological, biomechanical and anthropometrical predictors of sprint swimming performance in adolescent swimmers.' *Journal of Sports Science and Medicine* **9**(3):398–404.

219 Deschodt VJ, Arsac LM and Rouard AH (1999). 'Relative contribution of arms and legs in humans to propulsion in 25-m sprint front-crawl swimming.' *European Journal of Applied Physiology* 80(3): 192–9.

220 Counsilman JE (1968). The Science of Swimming. Prentice-Hall, Englewood Cliffs, NJ.

221 Fig, Grif (2005). Strength Training for Swimmers: Training the Core. *Strength & Conditioning Journal* **27**(10).

222 Santana JC (2003). The serape effect: A kinesiological model for core training. *Strength Cond. J.* **25**(2):73–4.

223 Santana J (2003). The Serape Effect: A kinesiological model for core training. *Strength and Conditioning Journal* **25**(2):73–4.

224 Brick NE, McElhinney MJ and Metcalfe RS (2018). 'The effects of facial expression and relaxation cues on movement economy, physiological, and perceptual responses during running.' *Psychology of Sport and Exercise* **34**:20–28.

225 Hamilton RJ, Paton CD and Hopkins WG (2006). 'Effect of high-intensity resistance training on performance of competitive distance runners.' *International Journal of Sports Physiology Performance* **1**(1):40–49.

226 Tipton M (2019). 'Drifting into unconsciousness: Jason Zirganos and the mystery of undetected hypothermia.' *British Journal of Sports Medicine* **53**(17):1047.

227 Saycell J, Lomax M, Massey H, et al. (2019). 'How cold is too cold? Establishing the lower water temperature limits for marathon swim racing.' *British Journal of Sports Medicine* **53**(17).

228 Tabata I, Nishimura K, Kouzaki M, Hirai Y, Ogita F, Miyachi M and Yamamoto K (1996). 'Effects of moderate-intensity endurance and high-intensity intermittent training on anaerobic capacity and VO2max.' *Medicine and Science in Sports and Exercise* **28**(10):1327–30.

229 Paton CD and Hopkins WG (2005). 'Combining explosive and high-resistance training improves performance in competitive cyclists.' *Journal of Strength and Conditioning Research* **19**(4):826–30.

230 Bishop D, Girard O and Mendez-Villanueva A (2011). 'Repeated-sprint ability – part II: recommendations for training.' *Sports Medicine* **41**(9):741–56.

231 McEwan G, Arthur R, Phillips SM, Gibson NV and Easton C (2018). 'Interval running with self-selected recovery: physiology, performance, and perception.' *European Journal of Sport Science* **18**(8): 1058–67.

232 Thomas C, et al. (2012). 'Effects of acute and chronic exercise on sarcolemmal MCT1 and MCT4 contents in human skeletal muscles: current status.' *American Journal of Physiology: Regulatory, Integrative and Comparative Physiology* **302**(1):R1–14.

233 Weston AR, Myburgh KH, Lindsay FH, Dennis SC, Noakes TD and Hawley JA (1997). 'Skeletal muscle buffering capacity and endurance performance after high-intensity interval training by well-trained cyclists.' *European Journal of Applied Physiology and Occupational Physiology* **75**(1):7–13.

234 Vikmoen O, Ellefsen S, Troen O, Hollan I, Hanestadhaugen M, Raastad T and Ronnestad BR (2016). 'Strength training improves cycling performance, fractional utilization of VO2max & cycling economy in female cyclists.' *Scandinavian Journal of Medicine and Science in Sport* **26**(4):384–96.

235 Kucia-Cztszczon K, Dybinkska E, Ambrozy T and Chwala W (2013). 'Factors determining swimming efficiency observed in less skilled swimmers.' *Acta of Bioengineering and Biomechanics* **15**(4): 115–24.

236 Vikmoen O, Ellefsen S, Troen O, Hollan I, Hanestadhaugen M, Raastad T and Ronnestad BR (2016). 'Strength training improves cycling performance, fractional utilization of VO2max and cycling economy in female cyclists.' *Scandinavian Journal of Medicine and Science in Sport* **26**(4):384–96.

237 Ronnestad BR, Hansen EA and Raastad T (2010). 'Effect of heavy strength training on thigh muscle cross-sectional area, performance determinants, and performance in well-trained cyclists.' *European Journal of Applied Physiology* **108**(5):965–75.

238 Lundberg TR, Fernandez-Gonzalo R, Tesch PA, Rullman E and Gustafsson T (2016). 'Aerobic exercise augments muscle transcriptome profile of resistance exercise.' *American Journal of Physiology* **310**(11):1279–87.

239 Ronnestad BR, Hansen EA and Raastad T (2011). 'Strength training improves 5-min all-out performance following 185 min of cycling.' *Scandinavian Journal of Medicine and Science in Sport* **21**(2):250–9.

240 Aagaard P and Andersen JL (2010). 'Effects of strength training on endurance capacity in top-level endurance athletes.' *Scandinavian Journal of Medicine and Science in Sport* **20**(Suppl. 2):39–47.

241 Bell GJ, Syrotuik DG, Attwood K and Quinney HA (1993). 'Maintenance of strength gains while performing endurance training in oarswomen.' *Canadian Journal of Applied Physiology* **18**(1):104–15.

242 Aktuğ Z, Vural S and Ibis S (2019). 'The effect of Theraband exercises on motor performance and swimming degree of young swimmers.' *Turkish Journal of Sport and Exercise* **21**(2):238–43.

243 Crowley E, Harrison A and Lyons M (2017). 'The impact of resistance training on swimming performance: a systematic review.' *Sports Medicine* **47**(11):2285–307.

244 Aspenes ST and Karlsen T (2012). 'Exercise-training intervention studies in competitive swimming.' *Sports Medicine* **42**(6):527–43.

245 Skucas K and Pokvytyte V (2018). 'Combined strength exercises on dry land and in the water to improve swimming parameters of athletes with paraplegia.' *Journal of Sports Medicine and Physical Fitness* **58**(3):197–203.

246 Anderson CE, Sforzo GA and Sigg JA (2008). 'The effects of combining elastic and free weight resistance on strength and power in athletes.' *Journal of Strength and Conditioning Research* **22**(2): 567–74.

247 Stevenson MW, Warpeha JM, Dietz CC, Giveans RM and Erdman AG (2010). 'Acute effects of elastic bands during the free-weight barbell back squat exercise on velocity, power, and force production.' *Journal of Strength and Conditioning Research* **24**(11): 2944–54.

248 Fig G (2005). 'Strength training for swimmers: training the core.' *Strength and Conditioning Journal* **27**(2):40–2.

249 Santana JC (2000). *The Essence of Stability Ball Training Companion Guide.* Cranston, RI: Perform Better, p. 205.

250 Beattie K, Kenny IC, Lyons M and Carson BP (2014). 'The effect of strength training on performance in endurance athletes.' *Sports Medicine* **44**(6):845–65.

251 Behm DG, Leonard AM, Young WB, Bonsey WA and MacKinnon SN (2005). 'Trunk muscle electromyographic activity with unstable and unilateral exercises.' *Journal of Strength and Conditioning* **19**(1):193–201.

252 Gutin B and Lipetz S (1971). 'An electromyographic investigation of the rectus abdominis in abdominal exercises.' *Research Quarterly for Exercise and Sport* **42**(3):256–63.

253 Phillips KC, Sassaman JM and Smoliga JM (2012). 'Optimizing rock climbing performance through sport-specific strength and conditioning.' *Strength and Conditioning Journal* **34**(3):1–18.

254 Macdonald JH and Callender N (2011). 'Athletic profile of highly accomplished boulderers.' *Wilderness and Environmental Medicine* **22**(2):140–3.

255 Ratamess NA, Faigenbaum AD, Mangine GT, Hoffman JR and Kang J (2007). 'Acute muscular strength assessment using free weight bars of different thickness.' *Journal of Strength and Conditioning Research* **21**(1):240–44.

256 Watts PB, Newbury V and Sulentic J (1996). 'Acute changes in hand-grip strength, endurance, and blood lactate with sustained sport rock climbing.' *Journal of Sports Medicine and Physical Fitness* **36**(4):255–60.

257 Watts PB, Daggett M, Gallagher P and Wilkins B (2000). 'Metabolic response during sport rock climbing and the effects of active

versus passive recovery.' *International Journal of Sports Medicine* **21**(3):185–90.

258 Watts PB (2004). 'Physiology of difficult rock climbing.' *European Journal of Applied Physiology* **91**(4):361–72.

259 Secomb JL, Farley ORL, Lundgren L, Tran TT, King A, Nimphius S and Sheppard JM (2015). 'Associations between the performance of scoring manoeuvres and lower-body strength and power in elite surfers.' *International journal of Sports Science & Coaching* **10**(5):911–18.

260 Turner A (2009). 'Training for power: principles and practice.' *Journal of Professional Strength and Conditioning* **14**:20–32.

261 Zatsiorsky V (1995). *Science and Practice of Strength Training.* Human Kinetics, Champaign, IL.

262 Kawamori N, Rossi SJ, Justice BD, Haff EE, Pistilli EE, O'Bryant HS, Stone MH, and Haff GG (2006). 'Peak force and rate of force development during isometric and dynamic mid-thigh clean pulls performed at various intensities.' *Journal of Strength and Conditioning Research* **20**(3):483–91.

263 Sheppard JM and Chapman DW (2011). 'An evaluation of strength qualities assessment for the lower body.' *Journal of Australian Strength and Conditioning* **19**(2):14–20.

264 Siff MC (2003). *Supertraining.* Supertraining Institute, Denver, CO.

265 Asci A and Acikada C (2007). 'Power production among different sports with similar maximum strength.' *Journal of Strength and Conditioning Research* **21**(1):10–16.

266 Baker D (2001). 'The effects of an in-season of concurrent training on the maintenance of maximal strength and power in professional and college-aged rugby league football players.' *Journal of Strength and Conditioning Research* **15**(2):172–7.

267 Aspenes ST and Karlsen T (2012). 'Exercise-training intervention studies in competitive swimming.' *Sports Medicine* **42**(6):527–43.

268 Stanley J, Peake JM, and Buchheit M (2013). 'Cardiac parasympathetic reactivation following exercise: implications for training prescription.' *Sport Medicine* **43**(12):1259–77.

269 Scott A. Heinlein, PT and Cosgarea AJ (2010). 'Biomechanical considerations in the competitive swimmer's shoulder.' *Sports Health* **2**(6):519–25.

270 Bak K (2010). 'The practical management of swimmer's painful shoulder: etiology, diagnosis, and treatment.' *Clinical Journal of Sport Medicine* **20**(5):386–90.

271 De Martino I and Rodeo SA (2018). 'The swimmer's shoulder: multi-directional instability.' *Current Reviews in Musculoskeletal Medicine* **11**(2):167–71.

272 Tovin BJ (2006). 'Prevention and treatment of swimmer's shoulder.' *North American Journal of Sports Physical Therapy* **1**(4):166–75.

273 Allegrucci M, Whitney SL and Irrgang JJ (1994). 'Clinical implications of secondary impingement of the shoulder in freestyle swimmers.' *Journal of Orthopaedic & Sports Physical Therapy* **20**(6): 307–18.

274 Matzkin E, Suslavich K and Wes D (2016). 'Swimmer's shoulder: painful shoulder in the competitive swimmer.' *Journal of the American Academy of Orthopaedic Surgeons* **24**(8):527–36.

275 Wilmore JH, Leon AS, Rao DC, Skinner JS, Gagnon J and Bouchard C (1997). 'Genetics, response to exercise, and risk factors: the HERITAGE Family Study.' *World Review of Nutrition and Dietetics* **81**:72–83.

276 Hubal M, Gordish-Dressman H, Thompson PD, Price TB, Hoffman EP, Angelopoulos TJ, Gordon PM, Moyna NM, Pescatello LS, Visich PS, Zoeller RF, Seip RL and Clarkson PM (2005). 'Variability in muscle size and strength gain after unilateral resistance training.' *Medicine and Science in Sport* **37**(6):964–72.

277 Beaven CM, Gill ND and Cook CJ (2008). 'Salivary testosterone and cortisol responses in professional rugby players after four resistance exercise protocols.' *Journal of Strength and Conditioning Research* **22**(2):426–3.

PART 3 | WHEN TO ADVENTURE

1 Jones KR, Klein CJ, Halpern BS, Venter O, Grantham H, Kuempel CD, Shumway N, Friedlander AM, Possingham HP and Watson JEM (2018). 'The location and protection status of earth's diminishing marine wilderness.' *Current Biology* **28**(15):2506–12

PART 4 | WHERE TO ADVENTURE

1 Knight DR and Horvath SM (1985). 'Urinary responses to cold temperature during water immersion.' *American Journal of Physiology: Regulatory, Integrative and Comparative Physiology* **248**(5):R560.

2 Wright DA, Sherman WM and Dernbach AR (1985). 'Carbohydrate feedings before, during, or in combination improve cycling endurance performance.' *Journal of Applied Physiology* **71**(3):1082–8.

6 Williams C, Brewer J and Walker M (1992). 'The effect of a high carbohydrate diet on running performance during a 30-km treadmill time trial.' *European Journal of Applied Physiology and Occupational Physiology* **65**(1):18–24.

4 Burke LM, Cox GR, Culmmings NK and Desbrow B (2001). 'Guidelines for daily carbohydrate intake: do athletes achieve them?' *Sports Medicine* **31**(4):267–99.

5 Balsom PD, Gaitanos GC, Söderlund K and Ekblom B (1999). 'High-intensity exercise and muscle glycogen availability in humans.' *Acta Physiologica Scandinavica* **165**(4):337–45.

6 Choi JS, Ahn DW, Choi JK, Kim KR and Park YS (1996). 'Thermal balance of man in water: prediction of deep body temperature change.' *Applied Human Science* **15**:161–7.

7 Holmer I and Bergh U (1974). 'Metabolic and thermal response to swimming in water at varying temperatures.' *Journal of Applied Physiology* **37**(5):702–5.

8 Tipton, M and Bradford C (2014). 'Moving in extreme environments: open water swimming in cold and warm water.' *Extreme Physiology & Medicine* **3**:12.

9 Nadel ER, Holmer I, Bergh U, Astrand PO and Stolwijk JA (1974). 'Energy exchanges of swimming man.' *Journal of Applied Physiology* **36**:465–71.

10 Vincent MJ and Tipton MJ (1988). 'The effects of cold immersion and hand protection on grip strength.' *Aviation Space and Environmental Medicine* **59**(8):738–41.

ACKNOWLEDGEMENTS

This book began as a set of incoherent 'sports science scribbles' in my training journal as I researched the damage caused by completing the World's Longest Sea Swim (1,780 miles around Great Britain) and studied ways to speed up my recovery so I could go from the surgery table back to the sea as fast as possible. But along the way it turned into something so much more, and that's only because of the incredible people I feel privileged to have met, coached, trained with and learned from.

This includes living legends of strength and conditioning whose feats are immortalised in 'fitness folklore' and detailed throughout the pages of this book, but (most importantly) it also involves two of the greatest training partners I could ever wish for, who so often operate behind the scenes. Supporting every one of my athletic adventures, Scott and Craig Edgley (better known as my brothers) have supported more miles at sea than I can count, and for this I am forever grateful.

Next, I need to thank my girlfriend, Hester Sabery. I've also lost count of the number of times you've helped put my bruised, battered and broken body back together (often with a freshly baked protein brownie and homemade ice cream). You're quite literally Superwoman and I think the main reason I attempt the impossible time and time again is because I know if I fail, you'll be there to catch me.

Finally, to the amazing publishing team at HarperCollins. Despite me arriving back on land after 157 days at sea in a urine-soaked wetsuit with parts of my tongue missing, you had faith in me as an author and shared my vision to create a book that would educate and empower millions. Which is why I'm forever grateful to everyone at HarperCollins HQ who's helped me publish and share with the world my philosophies and theories on strength and conditioning.

INDEX

Page references in *italics* indicate images.
RE indicates Ross Edgley.